T0259893

Advanced Practice Nursing Guide to the Neurological Exam

Alexandra Armitage, MS, APRN, CNL, is a clinical practitioner who has worked and taught in various clinical and educational neurological and neurosurgical settings. She received her BS from the University of Natal, South Africa, and her MS and post-master's APRN certificate from the University of New Hampshire. She is currently working as a provider at Neurosurgery of Southern New Hampshire in Nashua, New Hampshire. She has given numerous neurology and neurosurgical lectures to both nursing and nurse practitioner students and is keenly interested in advancing the neurological knowledge of all nurses. In addition, she is the book reviewer for the New Hampshire Nurse's Association. She is a member of Sigma Theta Tau and the American Academy of Neurology.

Advanced Practice Nursing Guide to the Neurological Exam

Alexandra Armitage, MS, APRN, CNL

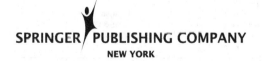

SPRINGER PUBLISHING COMPANY
NEW YORK

Springer Publishing Company, LLC
11 West 42nd Street
New York, NY 10036
www.springerpub.com

Acquisitions Editor: Margaret Zuccarini
Production Editor: Kris Parrish
Composition: S4Carlisle

ISBN: 978-0-8261-2608-5
e-book ISBN: 978-0-8261-2609-2

15 16 17 18 / 5 4 3 2 1

The author and the publisher of this Work have made every effort to use sources believed to be reliable to provide information that is accurate and compatible with the standards generally accepted at the time of publication. The author and publisher shall not be liable for any special, consequential, or exemplary damages resulting, in whole or in part, from the readers' use of, or reliance on, the information contained in this book. The publisher has no responsibility for the persistence or accuracy of URLs for external or third-party Internet websites referred to in this publication and does not guarantee that any content on such websites is, or will remain, accurate or appropriate.

Library of Congress Cataloging-in-Publication Data

Armitage, Alexandra, author.
  Advanced practice nursing guide to the neurological exam / Alexandra Armitage.
      p. ; cm.
  Includes bibliographical references and index.
  ISBN 978-0-8261-2608-5—ISBN 0-8261-2608-1—ISBN 978-0-8261-2609-2 (e-book)
  I. Title.
  [DNLM: 1. Neurologic Examination—nursing. 2. Nervous System Diseases—diagnosis. 3. Nursing Assessment. WY 160.5]
  RC386.6.N48
  616.8'0475—dc23
                                                                    2014043677

Printed in the United States of America by McNaughton & Gunn.

This book is dedicated to my wonderful husband, Graham, who has always been there for me, believing and encouraging me.

To my two marvelous children, Jason and Nicole, who light up my world.

To my mother, whose belief in the importance of education has been instrumental in my life.

And to my mentors over the years.

I could not have done it without you.

Contents

Preface   *ix*

PART I. INTRODUCTION TO THE BASIC NEUROLOGICAL EXAM

1. History Taking   *3*

2. Mental Status Testing   *11*

3. Cranial Nerves I and II   *21*

4. Cranial Nerves III, IV, and VI   *29*

5. Cranial Nerves V, VII, and VIII   *37*

6. Cranial Nerves IX, X, XI, and XII   *47*

7. Testing Motor Strength   *51*

8. Testing Sensation   *69*

9. Testing Reflexes   *79*

10. Balance and Gait   *91*

11. Testing Coordination   *105*

12. Imaging and EMG Studies   *113*

**PART II. COMMON NEUROLOGICAL SYMPTOMS AND CONDITIONS
        PRESENTED IN PRIMARY CARE**

13. Vertigo   *125*

14. Tremor   *141*

15. Low Back Pain   *151*

16. Peripheral Neuropathy   *171*

17. Weakness   *183*

18. Dementia   *197*

19. Diplopia   *207*

20. Gait Disturbance   *217*

21. Headache   *223*

Appendix: Useful Websites   *239*

Bibliography   *241*

Index   *245*

Preface

The majority of providers, including nurse practitioners, are often not comfortable with the assessment and diagnosis of the neurologic patient. It has been my observation that little time is spent on teaching neurology in nursing schools and as a result graduates tend to shy away from the initial assessment of the neurological patient.

Most neurological textbooks fall into one of two categories. The first group are brief and simplistic and do not provide the level of instruction required for practical application. The second group are tomes aimed primarily at those who already have a sound knowledge of neurology and neurological diseases. Their level of detail typically extends well beyond that of the primary clinic. In writing this book, my main motivation was to create the book that I wish had been available when I was new to the practice of neurology. It was important to me to write this book before I became too detached from the initial learning process and forgot the problems that posed the greatest challenges. The presentation of concepts in this book is a distillation of the education, mentoring, and self-study that surround my own growth in the neurological sciences.

When I first started in the field of neurology, I asked my mentor what was the most important thing for me to learn first. His response was, "Learn how to do an excellent neurologic examination." This advice has held me in good stead.

The information in this book is organized into two parts. The first part is dedicated to the neurological exam itself. It is my hope that the information provided will give you, the reader, a firm understanding of the preliminary assessment of the neurological patient, without feeling overwhelmed or intimidated. The second part of the book is dedicated to some of the more common symptoms that may be encountered in clinical practice. Understanding common etiologies, guidance on what questions and tests may be useful in an assessment of the disorder, and treatment options are detailed in these chapters.

It is my sincere hope that this book will empower you as a provider, and in doing so allow you to serve neurological patients better, both medically and empathetically. Patients arrive with symptoms that need to be placed in the context of a careful and detailed history and considered in light of the physical exam findings. In neurology, more than in many other disciplines, part of the practice is helping patients come to terms with what are often severe and debilitating illnesses for which sometimes there are few good treatments or cures. For this reason, establishing a good provider–patient relationship is important. In addition, staying in close contact with patients allows you to follow the natural course of the disease and gain a deeper understanding into the nature of the diagnosis. Finally, close follow-up will allow opportunities for reassessment, which will enable reconfirmation of the original diagnosis, thereby reducing the chances of perpetuating a misdiagnosis. I wish you much success and joy in the diagnosis, treatment, and continuing care of your neurological patients.

Alexandra Armitage

Introduction to the Basic Neurological Exam

I

History Taking

The most important part of an initial consultation with a patient is taking an accurate history. The history of present illness refers to the changes in health that have led the patient to seek medical care. It describes the information that is relevant to the patient's chief complaint. In taking an excellent history, the probable nature and probable site of the lesion may be deduced. This then guides the provisional diagnosis and subsequent physical exam, leading to a final definitive diagnosis and ultimately a treatment path.

■ ESSENTIAL ELEMENTS OF TAKING A GOOD HISTORY: LISTEN

The fundamental aspect of taking a good history is being a good listener. The patient should at all times feel as though he or she has your undivided attention regardless of how busy or rushed you are; the patient should not feel this pressure. For many patients being seen medically is a frightening experience, despite the fact that they may put on a brave face or act nonchalant. Being sensitive to this will help the patient relax and allow the patient to open up more easily and give a complete and accurate history. Every effort should be made to put the patient at ease. The successful interview is smooth and spontaneous. It is the process of establishing an extraordinary bond between patient and provider. On the basis of this trust, a patient will feel at ease to discuss intimate details of the illness. The establishment of such a relationship is steered by you, the interviewer. Not looking the patient in the eye, watching the clock, or interrupting the patient all undermine good communication with the patient. Spending a few minutes talking with the patient before the formal history taking and examination may serve to establish a rapport with the patient and to give you a better understanding of the patient's emotional state, mood, and intellectual capabilities. Once a rapport has been established with the patient, you should feel comfortable asking the patient any relevant, necessary questions, even sensitive ones. These questions must be easily understood by the patient, and language should be adjusted to the educational level and medical sophistication of the patient. If necessary, using informal slang words may facilitate communication. Once the patient is a little more at ease, the formal examination may begin with a discussion of actual symptoms.

■ FORMATTING THE HISTORY OF PRESENT ILLNESS

The patient's history of present illness may be organized using a consistent format, such as:

- Chief complaint including location, radiation, quality, and severity of symptoms
- Onset and precipitating event
- Associated symptoms
- Aggravating and relieving factors, including prior treatments
- Pertinent past medical and surgical history
- Occupational, psychosocial, and family history

THE CHIEF COMPLAINT

It is always important to ask the patient why he or she has come to the appointment; this will give an understanding of what the patient is hoping to get out of the encounter. It is not uncommon, for example, that a referral states that the patient is being referred for low back pain when in fact it is the neck that is bothering the patient more, or that the patient is being referred for neck pain when it is headaches that are most bothersome. In these cases, a clear understanding of what the patient is expecting, and having a discussion on what is being evaluated before the examination begins, is paramount. Once this has been established, begin by asking the patient about the actual symptoms that he or she is experiencing.

Hearing symptomology directly from the patient is important. Prior office notes from other providers that accompany the patient's referral may help guide questioning. However, don't just rely on these prior office notes, as this gives a secondhand account that has been screened by someone else and will not give a full patient history with the nuances that the patient may provide. Listening without interruption and allowing the patient to express himself or herself in his or her own words takes skill. The focus of history taking should be on the patient, and not the provider's agenda. When given the opportunity, patients will often reveal their own diagnosis spontaneously.

The art of listening is especially important with a patient who is a poor historian. It is not enough to simply state, "The patient is a poor historian"; this statement says as much about you, the examiner, as it does the patient. The questioning should be tailored to suit the patient. Learning to listen and then lead the interview with focused questions is an art that requires practice to perfect. Rushing the patient, in such cases, does nothing to aid the examination process, and may leave the patient feeling frustrated, unheard, and even angry.

In a similar manner, the patient who insists on telling every detail of the events remotely surrounding the situation can be even more challenging. In these cases, any effort to focus in on more specific points by specific questioning may lead to another whole string of irrelevant facts. There are times when you may have no choice but to politely stop the patient and refocus him or her on the issue at hand.

USE OPEN-ENDED QUESTIONS

The art of interviewing lies as much in the wording of the questions as in the body language and tone of voice used to ask it. In general, starting with an open-ended question is preferred as this allows the patient to talk freely about what is bothering him or her without presupposition.

Examples of open-ended questions include the following:

"What can I do for you today?"

"I understand that you have been having a lot of back pain. Can you tell me about it?"

Allow the patient to talk freely within reasonable boundaries. It may be necessary to refocus the patient—open-ended questioning is ill-advised with the overly talkative patient. After a period of open-ended talk, you can refocus the patient with direct questioning on points of interest that arose during the open-ended questioning.

USE DIRECT QUESTIONS

Direct questioning serves to clarify and add detail to the story. This type of questioning allows little room for the patient to add explanation:

"Show me where it hurts."

"Did the steroid taper you were given help you feel better?"

When asking direct questions, care must be taken not to ask leading questions.

However, often a patient does not know how to describe a symptom or is unwilling to volunteer more unusual symptoms for fear of judgment or being seen as irrational. In describing symptoms, it is acceptable, if needed, to give the patient a choice of adjectives to help him or her be more specific about what he or she is experiencing. This should be done in random order with no emphasis on any one particular descriptor. For example, if a patient complains of low back pain associated with leg pain, one may ask the patient whether the leg pain is in the front, side, or back of the leg or whether the pain encompasses the whole leg. Similarly, in describing this pain you may help the patient understand the kind of descriptors you are interested in by asking if the pain is sharp, shooting, burning, dull, throbbing, aching, electric, and so forth.

Using words that the patient can understand is as important as clarifying words that the patient chooses to use. If a patient describes his or her leg as numb, have the patient elaborate on this. Does he or she mean pins-and-needles or an anesthetic numbness? Avoid using technical words such as paresthesias and anesthesia. As the patient describes the symptoms, try and form a mental picture of how to tailor the physical examination to confirm what the patient is describing. Descriptions of bizarre symptoms should be noted and tested during the physical examination. This will allow you to understand the significance of the symptoms being described and determine whether there is evidence to support such claims.

MANAGE SENSITIVE ASPECTS OF SYMPTOMS

In some cases patients may not want to be completely open with their provider regarding the onset or nature of their symptoms owing to embarrassment or fear of judgment. This is especially true when the symptoms are related to subjects such as sexual activity, for example with exertional migraines. In these cases, it is necessary to tactfully but directly question the patient to get a clear picture of the sequence of events during the course of the history.

DETERMINING ONSET

To establish the beginning of the patient's complaint it is important to ascertain that the patient was completely well prior to the first sign. If this is an acute or chronic flare of a particular set of symptoms, understanding the patient's chronic baseline symptoms becomes important.

CROSS-CHECK

Cross-checking symptomology with a relative or friend can be very useful, and in some of the diseases that affect mentation can be absolutely vital to a meaningful assimilation of symptoms. If the patient wants to be accompanied to the appointment by someone, this should be welcomed and viewed as an opportunity to gain greater insight into the patient's complaints and help put him or her at ease with the whole examination. Ensure, however, that the patient is given the opportunity to talk, and is not completely overshadowed by his or her accompanying friend or relative. This is especially important if the patient does not speak English and the person accompanying the patient does. With foreign-language patients, one is obliged (and it is wise) to have a trained medical interpreter in the room to allow the patient the opportunity to communicate directly with you, through the interpreter, in his or her own words. In such cases, family members may add valuable information and insight into not only symptomology but the cultural differences that may exist; however, that should never replace listening directly to the patient. In some cases, such as early onset dementia, hearing certain symptomologic accounts from relatives can be very distressing for a patient. In addition, the family member may not be comfortable discussing these matters in front of the patient. In these cases, it may be better to interview the family members in another room, or the family member may be interviewed first, while the patient is in the waiting room prior to being welcomed into the examination room.

ASSOCIATED SYMPTOMS AND AGGRAVATING OR RELIEVING FACTORS

When questioning the patient, and as the differential diagnosis becomes clearer, ask about suspected associated symptoms. For example, if a patient is complaining of a unilateral headache and the description sounds like a migraine, you may ask the patient about nausea and vomiting, and light or sound sensitivity. Associated symptoms may help to confirm a diagnosis. What the patient describes is as important as what the patient does not describe. If a patient has a migraine but makes no mention of visual or other sensory disturbances, it is a good indication that the patient has not experienced an aura.

In a similar fashion, knowing what helps relieve or aggravate the patient's symptoms can narrow down the differential. In the previous example, a headache that is aggravated by light and sound serves to confirm the diagnosis of migraine. The effectiveness of particular medications that have been used in the past can also serve to confirm a diagnosis. Responsiveness of a headache to the use of triptans serves to further reinforce a migraine diagnosis. Another example would be a patient with a resting tremor who is suspected of having Parkinson's disease and who may have this diagnosis confirmed by responsiveness to levodopa.

PAST MEDICAL HISTORY

Obtaining a comprehensive past medical and surgical history is part of history taking. There are many medical and surgical conditions that have neurological implications. The neurological implications from diseases may either be directly from a condition, such as peripheral neuropathies in diabetes or AIDS; or by virtue of how the condition was treated, such as in the use of chemotherapeutic agents in cancer treatments leading to neuropathy or the use of antipsychotic agents for acute psychosis leading to tardive dyskinesia. Certain drugs, such as the antipsychotics, may have neurological side effects that present many years after taking them.

OCCUPATIONAL, PSYCHOSOCIAL, AND FAMILY HISTORY

INFLUENCE OF OCCUPATION

Occupation is important in understanding the chances that a patient was exposed to hazardous substances and understanding the physical requirements that the patient's job entails. Although these days exposure to hazardous substances is regulated much more tightly and is less of an issue than it was in the past, there is still a generation or two of patients that may have had considerable exposure to noxious substances. Understanding the physical requirements of the patient's job may explain the etiology of certain symptoms, such as backache in a patient who is required to do repetitive heavy lifting. It will also direct management and care of the patient, such as the use of a brace, or enrollment in a work-hardening physical therapy program. Occupation, like education, also gives insight into how functional the patient is in society and at what intellectual level one can expect to conduct the exam, answer further questions, and deliver subsequent explanations.

ALCOHOL, TOBACCO, AND ILLICIT (RECREATIONAL) DRUG USE

Alcohol, tobacco, and illicit (recreational) drug use should be determined as this may affect the physical exam findings. For example, the use of marijuana may significantly heighten a patient's reflexes. Use of these substances may also be a cause of neurological compromise such as in alcoholic cerebellar atrophy with resultant gait and balance disorders.

FAMILY HISTORY

Taking a careful family history is especially important in the consideration of heritable or environmental aspects of disease that might have implications for the patient. Determine the age and health of all immediate family members. When a disease has a late onset or the family has made efforts to cover up the existence of a disease in the family as a result of stigma, it can be tricky, but may also serve to confirm a diagnosis.

■ VALUE OF A THOROUGH PATIENT HISTORY

The true value of an excellent history becomes apparent when you prepare to do the physical exam as it allows you to tailor your examination to the patient. This is important as doing a full neurological exam on each patient would be time prohibitive and unnecessary. By the end of the patient's history taking you should have a very good idea of the patient's diagnosis. The history serves to guide the physical examination, indicating which aspects need to be done in detail. For example, the patient complaining of sudden changes in vision would not get the same examination as the patient who comes in with complaints of low back pain. This ability to tailor the physical exam is based solely on the patient history, which underscores its importance.

Having narrowed down the patient's complaints to a short list of differential diagnoses, you may move into the physical examination of the patient. This should be done in a manner that places the patient at ease. It is important to explain to the patient what you are about to do so that there are no surprises. Catching a patient off guard does not instill confidence or trust in you. Warning patients about aspects of the exam that may cause some discomfort or anxiety is advisable. Patients will withstand this discomfort more easily if it is spoken of ahead of time. For example, when doing pinprick testing, warn the patient that the pin is sharp, but the touch will be gentle and you will not break skin, and that all you want to know is whether the patient can feel the sharpness of the pin or not.

Not every patient that presents for evaluation has a neurological disease, or any disease at all for that matter. The longer the laundry list of complaints, the lower the probability that the patient has significant (or any) pathology. Often, it is the most self-effacing patients that have the gravest neurological findings. Nonetheless, every symptom that the patient mentions should be carefully considered.

■ SUMMARY

In neurology, more than in many other disciplines, part of the practice is helping the patient come to terms with what are often severe and debilitating illnesses, few of which have good treatment options. Establishing a good rapport with the patient from the start and serving as a support for him or her is important. In addition to the benefits to the patient, staying in close contact with the patient will allow you to follow the natural course of the disease and gain a deeper understanding into the nature of his or her diagnosis. Finally, close follow-up will allow opportunities for reassessment, which will allow for reconfirmation of the original diagnosis, thereby reducing the chances of perpetuating a misdiagnosis.

Mental Status Testing

Mental status evaluation includes testing of memory, orientation, intelligence, insight, and general health of the patient's psychic state. During the interview you will have already established a degree of insight into the mental status of the patient. You may have also been able to assess the patient's remote memory, affect, and judgment. The mental status exam involves a number of simple questions; a well-delivered examination is couched in such a way as to alleviate patient perceptions of these questions. However, when the questioning is too simplistic or repetitive, an open and direct explanation of testing may help secure patient participation.

There are a number of formal tests available for the assessment of mental status. Brief screening tests such as the Montreal Cognitive Assessment Test (MoCA), Mini-Mental State Examination (MMSE), or the 6-Item Cognitive Impairment Test (6CIT) are concise, structured to be comprehensive, and yield standardized scores. While all the exams are copyrighted, the MoCA and 6CIT exam are open to unrestricted clinical use. The original English version of the MoCA may be seen in Figure 2.1. There are two alternative/equivalent versions of the MoCA that should be used to decrease possible learning effects when the MoCA is administered repetitively, for example, every 3 months or less. In addition, it has been translated into more than 50 languages. The 6CIT (Table 2.1) uses six basic questions that assign a score for incorrect answers. This inverse score is then weighted to produce a total out of a possible 28. Scores of 0 to 7 are considered normal and 8 or more are considered significant. The test has both a high sensitivity and specificity even in mild dementia. The main disadvantage is the weighted scoring of the test, which can initially be confusing to the examiner; however, computer models have simplified this greatly. The MMSE has visuospatial, memory, delayed recall, and orientation questions very similar to the MoCA and the 6 CIT. The MMSE is only available commercially, and is subject to copyright infringement.

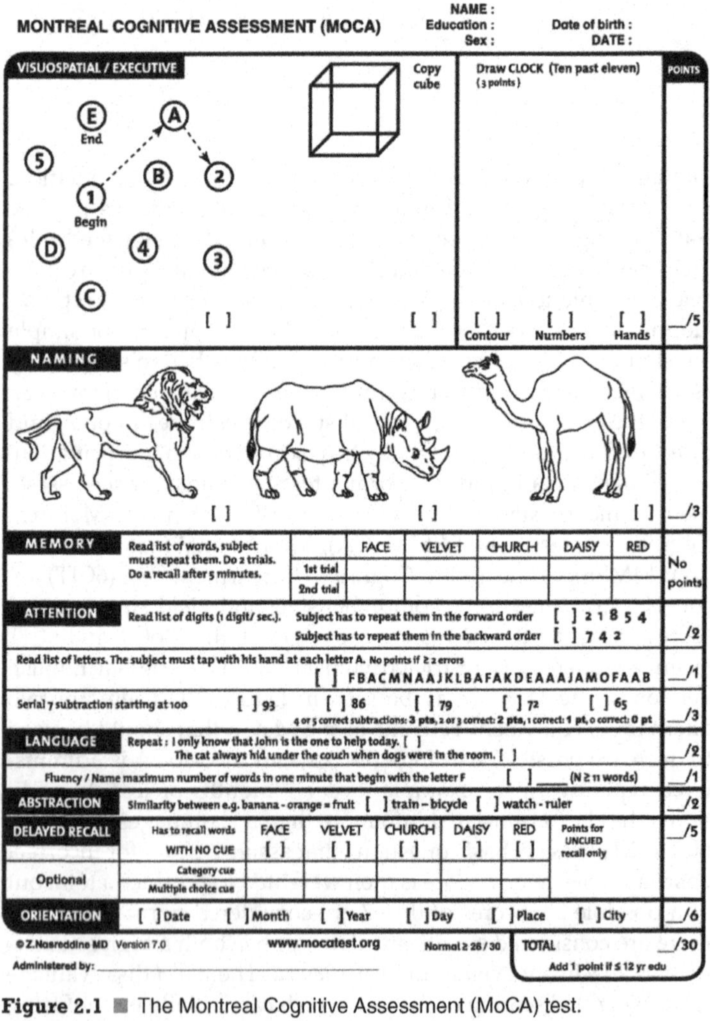

MONTREAL COGNITIVE ASSESSMENT (MOCA)

NAME :
Education :
Sex :
Date of birth :
DATE :

POINTS

VISUOSPATIAL / EXECUTIVE

E End, A, 5, B, 2, 1 Begin, D, 4, 3, C

[ ]

Copy cube [ ]

Draw CLOCK (Ten past eleven) (3 points)

[ ] Contour [ ] Numbers [ ] Hands ___/5

NAMING

[ ] [ ] [ ] ___/3

MEMORY

Read list of words, subject must repeat them. Do 2 trials. Do a recall after 5 minutes.

	FACE	VELVET	CHURCH	DAISY	RED
1st trial					
2nd trial					

No points

ATTENTION

Read list of digits (1 digit/ sec.). Subject has to repeat them in the forward order [ ] 2 1 8 5 4
Subject has to repeat them in the backward order [ ] 7 4 2 ___/2

Read list of letters. The subject must tap with his hand at each letter A. No points if ≥ 2 errors
[ ] FBACMNAAJKLBAFAKDEAAAJAMOFAAB ___/1

Serial 7 subtraction starting at 100 [ ] 93 [ ] 86 [ ] 79 [ ] 72 [ ] 65
4 or 5 correct subtractions: 3 pts, 2 or 3 correct: 2 pts, 1 correct: 1 pt, 0 correct: 0 pt ___/3

LANGUAGE

Repeat : I only know that John is the one to help today. [ ]
The cat always hid under the couch when dogs were in the room. [ ] ___/2

Fluency / Name maximum number of words in one minute that begin with the letter F [ ] ___ (N ≥ 11 words) ___/1

ABSTRACTION

Similarity between e.g. banana - orange = fruit [ ] train – bicycle [ ] watch - ruler ___/2

DELAYED RECALL

Has to recall words	FACE	VELVET	CHURCH	DAISY	RED	
WITH NO CUE	[ ]	[ ]	[ ]	[ ]	[ ]	Points for UNCUED recall only
Optional: Category cue						
Optional: Multiple choice cue						

___/5

ORIENTATION

[ ] Date [ ] Month [ ] Year [ ] Day [ ] Place [ ] City ___/6

© Z.Nasreddine MD Version 7.0 www.mocatest.org Normal ≥ 26 / 30 TOTAL ___/30
Administered by: ___ Add 1 point if ≤ 12 yr edu

Figure 2.1 ■ The Montreal Cognitive Assessment (MoCA) test. (Copyright Z. Nasreddine, MD. Reproduced with permission. Copies are available at www.mocatest.org.)

Table 2.1 ■ THE 6-ITEM COGNITIVE IMPAIRMENT TEST (6CIT)

Question	Score Range	Weighting	Weighted Score
What year is it?	0–1	×4	
What month is it?	0–1	×3	
Give the memory phrase (e.g., John/Smith/42/ West Street/ Bedford)	–	–	–
About what time is it?[1]	0–1	×3	
Count back from 20 to 1[2]	0–2	×2	
Say the months of the year in reverse[3]	0–2	×2	
Repeat the memory phrase[4]	0–5	×2	
Total score for 6CIT[5]	0–28		

[1]If the patient gets to within an hour of the correct time, then the patient scores zero; if not, score 1.

[2]One error = 1 point; 2 or more errors = 2 points (note they cannot score more than 2 for this question).

[3]One error = 1 point; 2 or more errors = 2 points (note they cannot score more than 2 for this question)

[4]Correct =0 points; 1 error =2 points; 2 errors =4 points; 3 errors = 6 points; 4 errors = 8 points; All wrong =10 points.

[5]0 to 7 = normal; 8–9 = mild cognitive impairment; 10 to 28 = significant cognitive impairment.

Source: Reproduced with kind permission of Dr. Patrick Brooke, The Kingshill Research Centre, Swindon, UK.

The numeric evaluation of a patient's mental status is of value if you want to compare testing outcomes over time or for providing consistency where there is more than one provider involved in the patient's care. Highly educated patients can score normally on these screening tests even in the presence of mild dementia. You need to be aware of the patient's age, education, and primary language as these may influence mental status test scores. All of these screening tests are quick to commit to memory and perform at the bedside. The specificity of the MoCA and 6CIT in screening for mild dementia is high, and they are neither sensitive to educational level nor dependent on advanced language skills, which make them valuable bedside tools.

Although overt signs and symptoms of psychiatric disturbance warrant a formal psychiatric evaluation, such a discussion is beyond the scope of this book.

■ ASSESSMENT OF LEVEL OF CONSCIOUSNESS

The level of consciousness can be assessed as soon as you introduce yourself to the patient. If the patient does not respond, take the patient's hand and repeat the introduction, asking the patient to squeeze your hand if he or she can hear you. If there is no response, try gently shaking the patient. If there is still no response, you can try and elicit a response by using a noxious stimulus such as applying pressure to the nail bed or a sternal rub. If these measures fail to rouse the patient, the patient is in a coma.

Level of consciousness may be assessed using a tool such as the Modified Glasgow Coma Scale (GCS). The GCS is a test that allocates a numeric value in a range of 3 to 15 (Table 2.2). Patients scoring 15 have no deficits; patients scoring 3 to 8 are said to be comatose. This tool provides an objective numeric value that allows serial evaluation of a patient across multiple providers. The GCS is now widely used among first responders and in the hospital setting.

■ ASSESSMENT OF SPEECH

During the first introductions, you will already have had the opportunity to assess the patient's speech. The patient may now be asked to repeat a short phrase such as "no ifs, ands, or buts."

Abnormalities of speech include dysphonia or aphonia, dysarthria or anarthria, and dysphasia or aphasia.

DYSPHONIA OR APHONIA

Dysphonia is the impairment of vocalization (phonation). Typically, the patient is hoarse; however, in extreme cases, vocalization

Table 2.2 ■ THE MODIFIED GLASGOW COMA SCALE

Assessment	Patient Response	Points
Eye-opening response	Spontaneous open with blinking at baseline	4
	To verbal stimuli, command, speech	3
	To pain only (not applied to face)	2
	No response	1
Verbal response	Oriented	5
	Confused conversation	4
	Inappropriate words	3
	Incomprehensible speech	2
	No response	1
Motor response	Obeys commands for movement	6
	Purposeful movement to painful stimulus	5
	Withdraws in response to pain	4
	Flexion in response to pain (decorticate posturing)	3
	Extension response in response to pain (decerebrate posturing)	2
	No response	1

is absent and the patient is mute. This complete loss of vocalization is known as aphonia.

The most frequent cause of this problem is the common cold, which results in dysphonia due to inflammation of the larynx. Neurological causes of dysphonia include damage to the recurrent laryngeal nerve and lesions of the vagus nerve. The recurrent laryngeal nerve may be damaged during neck surgery, such as in thyroidectomy or anterior cervical discectomy and fusion (ACDF) surgery. Intermittent hoarseness may affect patients with vagus nerve stimulator implants, which are used for the treatment of certain medically intractable forms of epilepsy and pharmacoresistant depression.

DYSARTHRIA OR ANARTHRIA

Dysarthria is the inability to articulate spoken words mechanically. The patient can understand the spoken word and is able to formulate a coherent response, but is unable to form the spoken words effectively. The presentation typically is slurred speech. Anarthria is when there is a complete lack of ability to articulate words.

The pharyngeal, palatal, lingual, or facial musculatures are commonly involved, but these abnormalities may also be seen with certain cerebellar lesions.

DYSPHASIA OR APHASIA

Aphasia is a breakdown in the synthesis of language, with dysphasia representing a partial breakdown of this process. Aphasia may be a result of breakdown in any or all of three processes. It may present as an inability (a) to understand written or spoken language (known as receptive, sensory, or Wernicke aphasia), (b) transfer signals from the Wernicke to the Broca area (conduction aphasia), or (c) properly formulate speech (expressive, motor, or Broca aphasia). The combination of Wernicke and Broca aphasias results in an inability either to comprehend or formulate speech and is referred to as global aphasia.

■ ASSESSMENT OF ORIENTATION

Orientation is an individual's awareness of self in relation to time, place, and person. Generally, the sense of time is the first to be impaired in organic dysfunction, and the sense of person is the last to be lost. However, the order may be disturbed in psychological dysfunction.

The patient should be able to state his or her name and birthdate, give today's date and day of the week, and know the name of the hospital or building that he or she is currently in.

ORIENTATION TO PERSONS

Open up the conversation by asking the patient his or her name. As stated, this is the last function to be lost. Patients who have almost complete white matter "white-outs" from anoxic injury and who cannot even feed themselves still may be able to answer this question.

Now pointing to a friend or relative who is with the patient, you can ask, "Who is this?" Close family, such as children, are almost always remembered. Grandchildren and friends, however, add a more impartial determination.

ORIENTATION TO PLACE

Basic questions include, "Where are we?" "What floor are we on?" (outpatient only), or "What building are we in?"

Work in a specific to general fashion: "What [city, state, county]?" Remember to be realistic: If the patient is not native to the area, try asking about where he or she lives, such as an address, where he or she works, what state he or she comes from, his or her telephone number. You do not need to ask all of these questions; tailor it to the patient you are currently assessing.

ORIENTATION TO TIME/DATE/SEASON

These questions are more straightforward: "What is today's date [month, year]?" "What day of the week is it?" "What season is it?" If there has been a major holiday recently or one coming up, you can ask the patient if he or she can name it for you. This is an interesting set of questions as they are sensitive but not always very specific. Make sure that there is no large, well-displayed calendar behind you as you ask the question!

■ ASSESSMENT OF MEMORY

Memory is the ability to register and recall prior events. Recent and remote memory functions are affected differently depending on the disease process. Remote memory is the last to be lost in chronic dementing processes, with major disturbances in the attention span and recent memory. On the contrary, all aspects of memory are impaired in acute encephalopathies.

To test remote memory, have the patient recall well-known events from the past. Do not ask about things that you cannot verify. More recent memory is most easily tested by asking the patient about current events, aspects of the patient's current situation (e.g., "What did you eat for breakfast today?"), or giving the patient three things to remember; for example, "cat, baseball, Chevrolet."

IMMEDIATE RECALL

Immediate memory is tested by asking the patient to remember a set of items and recount them in an immediate time frame, first without and then with distraction. "Remember these three things for me: rose, ball, house." Have the patient repeat the three things: Most patients can do this without coaching. Patients get no points for being able to repeat the words immediately, but it is telling if they require considerable coaching to get to the point of repetition.

After 5 minutes of distraction with other test questions, ask the patient what those initial three things were, give them a minute, and allow them to remember them in any order they choose.

There is no point in belaboring the issue. If they have not been able to remember, you may choose to give them clues (such as "one item is a flower"). Regardless, the patient gets no credit from a diagnostic point of view; however, this is the task that patients who are being evaluated for cognitive issues are most sensitive to. Patients should never be made to feel as if they have failed at this task.

ABILITY TO RECOUNT VERY RECENT EVENTS

The ability to recount recent events may be tested through a variety of ways, and generally two or perhaps three questions are all that it takes to get a good sense of whether there is an issue here.

"What did you have for breakfast?" (Make sure you know or are with someone who does.)

"Do you read? How well can you remember what you read? When you get to the bottom of the page, can you remember what you read from the top of the page?" (Not only is it fairly common for a person with memory problems to find this an issue, but it is almost never found in people who do not have cognitive issues.)

Ask the patient to describe the types of things that he or she typically forgets, such as difficulty finding keys, accidentally leaving the stove on, or remembering the reason he or she walked into a room. All of the above are (very) commonly found in cognitively intact people. There is the adage that it is not so important if you forget why you are going up or down the stairs, but it is quite telling if you stop in the middle of the stairs and then forget whether you were going up or down.

Remembering food choices at meals, the ability to retain read information over a short period of time, and the number of sticky notes or lists that a person requires to be able to continue with his or her normal activities of daily living are the most useful questions as they are typically intact in normal folk and reasonably objective in nature.

ASSESSMENT OF LONG-TERM MEMORY

Ability to recall past events may be evaluated by asking patients where they were born, where they grew up, and how many children they have. Remember that if you do not know the correct answer, your question is pointless. Many a demented patient answers these questions very confidently and without pause, all the while confabulating the answers.

Little time is spent on this in clinical practice because, like remembering one's name, a patient loses long-term memory function last.

■ ASSESSMENT OF ABSTRACT REASONING

Abstraction is a higher cerebral function that requires both comprehension and judgment. Interpretation of proverbs tends to be used routinely to judge abstract reasoning. An example of such proverbs is "People in glass houses should not throw stones."

An appropriate answer would be "The proverb means that you should not criticize other people for bad qualities in their character that you have yourself." A literal or concrete answer may be something like "Stones can cause glass to break." A literal interpretation of the proverb may be expected from patients with certain organic or psychiatric mental disease.

Proverbs, however, have the disadvantage of being weighted heavily in favor of those with a good memory and superior schooling. When using proverbs, caution should be used when assessing patients whose mother tongue is not English.

Asking a patient to explain similarities between pairs (e.g., table–chair, ship–horse, poem–statue, watch–ruler) does not rely on either schooling or memory and is, therefore, preferable.

■ ASSESSMENT OF GENERAL FUND OF KNOWLEDGE

The patient's fund of knowledge is a function of his or her education and life experiences. In dementia, a patient's loss of knowledge is very telling. It is helpful to know the patient's highest educational level and the patient's occupation to be able to assess roughly how sophisticated a question he or she should be able to answer. A refugee with no high school education and a different culture should not be penalized for lack of breadth and depth in understanding American culture or knowledge base. Similarly, if a well-educated patient is concerned about cognitive decline, asking a set of simple questions is not going to elucidate the answer.

■ ASSESSMENT OF CALCULATION

The ability to calculate depends on the integrity of the dominant cerebral hemisphere, the patient's intelligence, and the patient's schooling. Counting serial 3s, serially subtracting 7 starting at 100, or basic addition all serve well to assess a patient's competence with calculation.

■ ASSESSMENT OF OBJECT RECOGNITION

Agnosia is the failure of a patient to recognize an object despite normal vision. Show the patient well-known objects such as a pen, a ruler, a wristwatch, or glasses, and ask the patient to name them. If the patient has normal vision but is unable to name the object, the patient has visual agnosia. Tactile agnosia is the inability of a patient to recognize an object by palpation in the absence of a sensory deficit.

■ ASSESSMENT OF VOLUNTARY MOVEMENT

Apraxia is the inability to perform a voluntary movement despite intact motor strength, sensation, and coordination. Ask a patient to do a voluntary task, such as brushing the hair. The patient hears and understands the request, but is unable to integrate the motor activities required to complete the activity. When a patient cannot construct a representation of an object on paper, it is known as constructional apraxia. Ask the patient to copy a drawing you have made or place numbers and hands of a given time onto the face of a clock.

Cranial Nerves I and II

Afferent nerves are special sensory nerves that carry sensory signals to the brain. Efferent nerves are special motor nerves that carry motor signals from the brain to the target location, such as a muscle group.

■ CRANIAL NERVE I: OLFACTORY NERVE

Cranial nerve (CN) I is a special sensory (afferent) nerve for smell. Damage to the olfactory nerve leads to a reduced ability to taste and smell. The inability to smell from damage to the olfactory nerve may be tested by having a patient smell a nonirritating and familiar-smelling substance. Testing requires the patient to close one nostril and his or her eyes and then sniff the substance and identify it. The procedure is repeated for the other side. If the patient can identify the smell presented, it is assumed that the olfactory tract is intact. Suitable substances would include coffee grounds, vanilla, banana, peppermint, or chocolate. Ammonia to test the olfactory nerve is inappropriate as it is caustic to the mucosa and irritating to the free nerve ending, which may cause pain and elicit a pain response. Lesions of the olfactory nerve do not affect the ability of the nasal epithelium to sense pain. This is because pain from the nasal epithelium is carried to the central nervous system via the trigeminal nerve (CN V) and not the olfactory nerve.

Although testing of CN I is quick and easy, it is seldom included as part of the bedside test or office consult. Defects in olfaction may be indicative of anterior skull base tumors, blunt trauma such as coup-contrecoup damage, and meningitis. The incidence of olfactory deficit in traumatic brain injury (TBI) is directly related to the severity of trauma. This deficit is also commonly correlated with the presence of cognitive impairment following TBI. It has been suggested that deficits in olfaction may be used as an objective marker of persistence of TBI in patients that are otherwise neurologically intact. Neurodegenerative conditions such as Alzheimer's and Parkinson's disease may also present with olfactory dysfunction, often in the prodromal period prior to the presentation of other overt symptomology.

■ CRANIAL NERVE II: OPTIC NERVE

CN II is the sensory (afferent) nerve of vision. The visual field is defined as everything one can see without moving one's head.

PUPILLARY LIGHT REFLEX

The pupillary light reflex allows the eye to adjust to various light intensities by changing pupil size with changing light levels. A complete pupillary reflex requires detection of the light (CN II–afferent nerves) that is relayed to the brainstem. The response is relayed back to both eyes according to the light level by dilation or contraction or the constrictor pupillae muscles in the iris (CN III–efferent nerve.) This is a brainstem-mediated reflex that does not involve the cerebral cortex.

The pupillary light reflex is elicited by shining a light into a patient's eye. A normal response is the constriction of the pupils in both eyes: the eye where the light was shone (direct light reflex) and the eye that did not have the light shone in it (consensual light reflex). Both pupils should constrict equally without evidence of pupillary redilation when a flashlight is swung backward and forward from one eye to another (the "swinging flashlight test"). You may notice hippus in some patients when examining their eyes. Hippus refers to nonrhythmic fluctuations in pupillary size when there is a steady illumination; this is a benign phenomenon and is considered a variant of normal.

The neural pathway that manages the afferent pupillary reflex runs directly to the midbrain for the sole purpose of light detection to protect the sensitive retina from excess light. The presence of this reflex is one of the most basic tests of brainstem function, and is one of the reflexes tested in determining brain death.

AFFERENT PUPILLARY DEFECT

Damage to the optic nerve in one eye causes an afferent pupillary defect, which is an important clinical finding. The most effective test for this in a clinical setting is to slightly darken a room (especially if the patient has dark eyes) and then swing a light from eye to eye. Light shone into the normal eye will cause constriction of both pupils whereas light shone into the defective eye will not, as light detection in the damaged eye is reduced due to damage to the optic nerve. So swinging the flashlight back and forth between eyes will show bilateral pupillary constriction with light shone in the good eye and then apparent dilation of the pupils with light into the damaged eye. This apparent dilation is simply a response to removal of the light from the normal eye and the defective eye not detecting light as well as it should. Optic neuritis is overwhelmingly the most common cause of an afferent pupillary defect, and it has serious pathologic implications, with multiple sclerosis and neuromyelitis optica being at the top of the differential diagnosis list.

VISUAL FIELDS

The second cranial nerve carries visual signals from the retina to the occipital cortex. Compression or damage to CN II will cause defects in or loss of vision. Lesions along the visual pathway will cause visual defects that will vary depending on the location of the injury. In Figure 3.1, visual field defects along the visual pathways are depicted. Circles indicate what the left and right eyes see. Black areas represent visual field defects.

Peripheral vision field testing at the bedside or in the outpatient clinic is tested by confrontation. Have the patient cover one eye and instruct him or her to look at your nose. Flash or wiggle fingers in the patient's peripheral field of vision and ask the patient how many fingers are being displayed or which finger is wiggling. Using the limits of your own visual field enables you to test whether the patient has the same extent of visual field (Figure 3.2). If there is any doubt or if the findings are subtle, a formal field of vision testing should be done by an ophthalmologist. Peripheral vision may decrease in migraine with aura events, patients with cataracts, patients with lesions at various parts of the optic tract, or patients with eye defects.

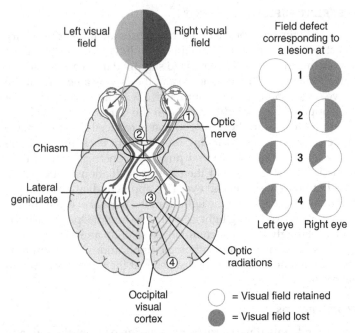

Figure 3.1 ■ The visual pathways as seen from above the brain.

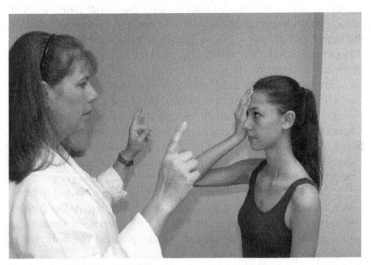

Figure 3.2 ■ Peripheral field testing.

It is important to realize that a narrowing of the visual field or a loss of the visual field in one quadrant is significantly different from an acute loss of sight from the top down, best described as a black curtain descending over an eye, in a top to bottom–like fashion. Loss of vision that occurs acutely as a curtain coming down over generally one eye (but perhaps two eyes) is known as amaurosis fugax, and it is a medical emergency. The most common and most devastating cause of such vision loss is carotid dissection, which needs to be ruled out immediately.

VISUAL ACUITY

Visual acuity is tested with a Snellen chart. The patient stands 20 feet from the chart. The chart consists of a series of symbols, for example, block letters, in gradually decreasing sizes (Figure 3.3). The visual acuity is stated as a fraction: the distance from the chart, 20 feet, is the numerator; the distance at which a "normal eye" would be able to read the last line that the patient is able to read is the denominator. For example, 20/20 vision signifies normal vision, that is, a patient can read a line of symbols at 20 feet that a person with "normal visual acuity" would be able to read at 20 feet. A person with poor vision may have, for example, 20/40 vision, that is, they are able to read at 20 feet what a person with normal vision can read at 40 feet. A person with better than normal vision will have a denominator that is less than 20, for example, if their score is 20/15, this person can read at 20 feet what a person with normal visual acuity can only read at 15 feet. At 20/200, a person is considered legally blind if they cannot read the 20-foot line, even with their best corrective lenses. Bedside testing of visual acuity may be done with a handheld Snellen chart, which is scaled to be held at comfortable arm's length.

THE FUNDOSCOPIC EXAM

The fundoscopic exam is a skill developed with practice. Looking into the eye at the disc, fovea, and retinal surface is an important part of the neurological exam. This is one of the most frustrating skills to learn as it takes time, patience, and skill, not to mention a willing patient. It is worth the effort and may allow the detection of urgent and emergent pathologies in a timely fashion. Table 3.1 outlines some of the common findings on exam with common causes for these findings. It should be remembered that papilledema does

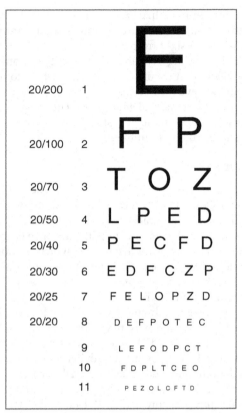

Figure 3.3 ■ Snellen chart for visual acuity testing.

not present in acute head injury as it takes 10 to 14 days to develop. It is the hallmark of chronic raised intracranial pressure or chronic optic disc pathology.

Of course, having a good look into the posterior chamber of a patient's eye takes practice. Cataracts and contact lenses complicate the endeavor. You may ask the patient to remove contact lenses if need be. It is also not uncommon to get a light shine-back secondary to your eyes focusing on the anterior and not the posterior of the eye. This can be worked through by using the ophthalmoscope to look at the patient's eye from a distance, focusing on the pink retinal area, and then slowly moving closer to the eye until the retina and the optic disc are clearly visualized. Cataract

Table 3.1 ■ KEY SIGNS IN A FUNDOSCOPIC EXAM

Change Seen	Interpretation	Possible Etiologies
Papilledema (blurred disc margins/loss of visible venous pulsations)	Increased intracranial pressure	Hydrocephalus, intracranial mass effect from a lesion, idiopathic intracranial hypertension
Disc pallor	Optic atrophy (either acute or chronic)	Multiple sclerosis
		Neuromyelitis optica
Excessive disc cupping	Increase intraocular pressure	Glaucoma
Microaneurysms	Increased small capillary pressure	Chronic hypertension, diabetic retinopathy
Macular edema	Blood vessels leak contents into the macular region	Diabetic retinopathy

surgery will render a patient's eyes pseudophakic and make visualization of the optic disc and fovea more difficult. When looking for venous pulsation, keep a hand on the patient's radial pulse for correlation.

COLOR DESATURATION

Color desaturation testing may be done as simply as asking the patient about color differences between eyes, using a red-colored object (tip of a reflex hammer or small red-tipped pencil) one eye at a time. This test detects subtle differences in the function of the optic nerve.

Cranial Nerves III, IV, and VI

4

Cranial nerves (CN) III, IV, and VI are motor (efferent) nerves that control the six muscles of the eye (three pairs of antagonistic muscles). CN VI innervates the lateral rectus muscle, while CN IV innervates the superior oblique muscle. CN III innervates the other four extraocular muscles: the medial rectus, inferior rectus, superior rectus, and inferior oblique (Figure 4.1). In addition, CN III controls the muscles that allow the pupils to constrict or dilate and the muscle above the eye known as the levator palpebrae superioris muscle, which elevates the eyelid.

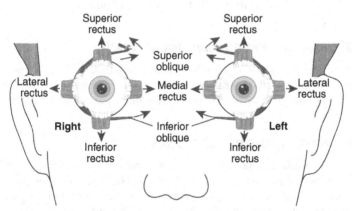

Figure 4.1 ■ Muscles responsible for the movement of the eyes.

■ CRANIAL NERVE III: OCULOMOTOR NERVE

CN III plays a major role in eye movement. It innervates four of the six extraocular eye muscles. It also innervates the muscle that elevates the upper eyelid (levator palpebrae superioris muscle). These are the somatic motor components of CN III. In addition, it innervates muscles that control the shape of the lens and size of the pupils (the constrictor pupillae and ciliary muscles), which form the visceral motor (parasympathetic efferent) component of CN III. The parasympathetic and somatic axons together form CN III with the parasympathetic axons surrounding the somatic motor axons. The fibers run from the midbrain, maintaining their special relationship all the way to their entry into the orbit, where they break out to innervate their respective musculature.

■ CRANIAL NERVE IV: TROCHLEAR NERVE

The trochlear nerve, CN IV, is the smallest of the cranial nerves and innervates only a single muscle—the superior oblique muscle. It has only a somatic motor component, which is intorsion of the eye and downward gaze. The initial position of the eye determines the eye movement effected by the superior oblique muscle.

■ CRANIAL NERVE VI: ABDUCENS NERVE

The abducens nerve, CN VI, like its counterpart CN IV, innervates only one muscle, the lateral rectus muscle. It is a somatic motor nerve with the sole function of moving the eye laterally away from midline.

■ CN III, IV, AND VI NERVE PALSY

The six muscles that control eye movement are innervated by three cranial nerves: CN III, IV, and VI. These six muscles form three yoked pairs of muscles. When one of the muscles in the pair contracts, the other relaxes. Upward, downward, and lateral eye gazes are controlled by four of the six extraocular eye muscles. The remaining two muscles control intorsion and extorsion of the eye. Figure 4.2 depicts extraocular eye movements in the cardinal positions of gaze. In conjunction with each other, these six muscles serve to keep the eye position stable and to track smoothly.

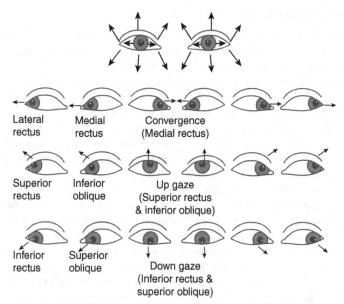

Figure 4.2 ■ Yoked extraocular eye movements in cardinal positions of gaze.

Lack of function of a nerve is known as a palsy. Cranial nerve palsies may be congenital or acquired later in life as a result of trauma, infection, or vascular disease. The primary presenting symptom when there is recent damage to CN III, IV, and VI is diplopia (double vision), as the eye muscle is not innervated correctly, causing weakness. If a muscle in one eye is weak, that eye cannot move smoothly in concert with the other healthy eye, causing disconjugate gaze (both eyes not focusing on the same object). Gazing in directions controlled by the weak muscle, which results in a disconjugate gaze, causes the patient to experience diplopia. The direction of gaze for which a patient experiences diplopia will depend on which cranial nerve is affected. Although innervated by three cranial nerves, eye movements are tested together.

A cranial nerve may have a complete or partial palsy. In a cranial nerve that has multiple functions, such as CN III, it is possible for a palsy to affect just some or all of the various functions of that nerve. The vascular diseases that most commonly affect the eye include diabetes, hypertension, strokes, and aneurysms.

THIRD NERVE PALSY

Damage to the third cranial nerve may affect some or all of the functioning of these muscles (Table 4.1). The parasympathetic axons are responsible for pupil constriction and lens shape (accommodation); they encircle the motor axons that serve the extraocular muscles and the levator palpebrae superioris muscle. When the nerve is compressed, the parasympathetic component is affected first. Infarction of the nerve, however, will affect the somatic motor component first, as these axons run through the center of the nerve. Damage to the somatic motor axons of the third nerve affects all targeted muscles.

A CN III lesion results in ipsilateral ptosis (eyelid droop) due to inactivation of the levator palpebrae superioris muscle, a dilated and unresponsive pupil due to reduced tone in the constrictor pupillae muscle, and an eye that looks down and out due to unopposed action of the superior oblique and lateral rectus muscles (Figure 4.3). The patient will have an inability to focus both eyes on the same object, resulting in double vision, although this may not be the patient's first complaint as the ptosis covers one eye.

Most third nerve palsies are due to ischemic events commonly caused by diabetes or hypertension. It is important not to miss an aneurysm pressing on the third nerve, and involvement of the parasympathetic component of CN III, presenting as a blown pupil, should be considered a medical emergency until proven otherwise. MRI and angiography are warranted to rule out aneurysm or tumor.

THE PUPILLARY REFLEX

Pupillary action and reaction involve testing CN III in conjunction with CN II, which forms the pupillary light reflex as discussed previously. CN II is responsible for the light detection portion of the pupillary reflex (afferent). CN III is responsible for the muscle reaction to this detection of light (efferent). In this reflex, a constriction of the pupils in both eyes is elicited by shining a light into one of the patient's eyes (see CN II pupillary light reflex).

When shining a light into an eye that has a CN III defect, the pupil will not react (constrict) to light despite the fact that the light is detected by CN II. The consensual pupil that has intact CN III enervation will react. Simply put, the eye can detect the light but cannot react to the light as the nerves to the muscles are damaged.

Table 4.1 ■ EXAM FINDINGS INVOLVING THE THIRD CRANIAL NERVE

Defect Observed on Physical Exam	Etiology	Mechanism	Example of Pathology
No pupil constriction in one eye with exposure to light. Direct and consensual pupil constriction in the other eye	Defect of parasympathetic axons of CN III	Pressure on the exterior of the CN III nerve	Tumor, aneurysm, inflammation, infection, or thrombosis exerting pressure on CN III
No pupil constriction in one eye with exposure to light	Complete CN III lesion on the affected side	Ischemic injury, infarction, or trauma to CN III lesion	Third nerve palsy
Direct and consensual pupil constriction in the other eye			
Ptosis			
Downward abduction of the affected eye			
Inability to accommodate			
Pupil constriction with abnormal CN III muscle movement	CN III extraocular eye musculature	Ischemic injury or infarction to the somatic motor axons of CN III	Diabetes, hypertension
Inability to intort and impaired downward gaze in the affected eye	CN IV	Congenital, trauma, ischemic injury, or infarction due to diabetes, hypertension	Fourth nerve palsy
Abduction defect in affected eye	CN VI	Tumor, infection, or infarction commonly due to diabetes, hypertension	Sixth nerve palsy

CN, cranial nerve.

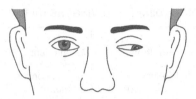

Figure 4.3 ■ Third nerve palsy demonstrating ptosis (eyelid droop) due to inactivation on the levator palpebrae superioris muscle, a dilated and unresponsive pupil due to reduced tone in the constrictor pupillae muscle, and an eye that looks down and out due to unopposed action of the superior oblique and lateral rectus muscles.

EXTRAOCULAR EYE MOVEMENT AND VISUAL FIELDS TESTING

Stand in front of the patient and ask the patient to follow your finger with the eyes only. In the air before the patient, slowly draw a box or an H-shape in the air. Ask the patient to report any loss of vision or diplopia while you are doing this. While you are doing this, observe the patient for nystagmus. Nystagmus is an oscillation of the eyes and may be vertical or horizontal. The eyes should track with smooth coordination. The presence of nystagmus may be normal or indicative of pathology. Some patients have congenital nystagmus. Remarkably, this can be quite severe, and yet the patients do not complain of vision problems as they have adjusted to these rapid eye movements.

FOURTH NERVE PALSY

When a superior oblique muscle stops functioning, the inferior oblique extorts and slightly elevates the eye. This lack of concordance between the eyes results in the image projected onto different areas of the right and left retinas, which results in two distinct images being seen (diplopia). The images are seen vertically and slightly to one side from each other. A palsy of the trochlear nerve leaves the affected eye rotated up and in, because the action of the superior oblique muscle is to rotate the eye down and out (Figure 4.4). Tilting the head away from the dysfunctional side may improve the patient's vision by obliging the opposite side to intort, thereby compensating. Some people develop a paradoxical head tilt toward the side of the lesion, which amplifies the discrepancy between the two images, allowing them to ignore one of them.

A fourth nerve palsy can be very difficult to detect, and observing the downward gaze when the eye is adducted may be the most sensitive test. Fourth nerve lesions can be caused by trauma, ischemia, tumor, or they may be congenital. Ischemic events are most commonly from diabetes or hypertension.

SIXTH NERVE PALSY

A patient with a sixth nerve palsy will have double vision when looking at an object on the same side as the lesion (Figure 4.5), but when looking away from the lesion, the double vision will resolve.

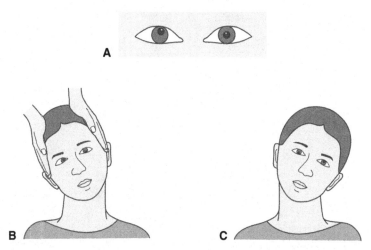

Figure 4.4 ■ Fourth nerve palsy. (A) Straight-ahead gaze with the affected eye rotated up and in; (B) head tilted towards the lesion causes the greatest divergence of symptoms; and (C) head tilted to the unaffected side corrects the vision defect.

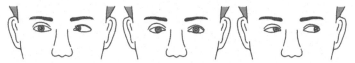

Figure 4.5 ■ Sixth nerve palsy of the right eye.

Cranial Nerves V, VII, and VIII

5

■ CRANIAL NERVE V: TRIGEMINAL NERVE

Cranial nerve (CN) V is best known as the nerve that supplies the brain with sensory input from the face. CN V, however, has both sensory and motor functions. The fifth cranial nerve is divided into three branches. All three divisions of the fifth cranial nerve contain sensory nerve fibers. The third division (mandibular, V3) has both sensory and motor (afferent and efferent) fibers.

The first division of CN V innervates the forehead (ophthalmic, V1) and as far back as the coronal suture (Figure 5.1).

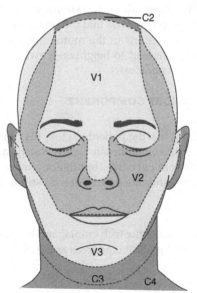

Figure 5.1 ■ V1, V2, and V3 dermatomal divisions of CN V.

V1 is the only division of CN V that is bilaterally innervated, and therefore sensation or sensory changes are never unilateral. This is important to know when testing a patient as it is one of the ways to tease out true sensory loss from functional symptomatology.

The second division of CN V innervates the area from the ear to the maxilla (maxillary, V2). The third portion innervates the mandible and lower structures of the face (mandibular, V3). V2 and V3 are innervated unilaterally—that is, the left-sided nerve branch innervates the left side of the face, and the right-sided nerve branch innervates the right side of the face. V3 is the only division that has both sensory and motor fibers. The motor fibers of V3 have bilateral cortical representation and are involved in chewing, biting, and swallowing. Because of this bilateral representation, a central lesion (e.g., a stroke) *will not* produce any observable deficit. In contrast, a peripheral nerve injury will cause paralysis of muscles on one side of the jaw, resulting in the jaw deviating to the paralyzed side when it opens.

The motor component of V3 also innervates the tensor tympani muscle in the middle ear. The tensor tympani muscle helps to dampen sound in the ear by tightening the tympanic membrane and reducing the amplitude of the sound wave that gets transmitted to the ossicles. The noise that it dampens is predominantly sounds of chewing. Lesions in the motor component of the fifth cranial nerve (V3) can lead to heightened awareness of chewing sounds (a form of hyperacusis).

TESTING THE SENSORY COMPONENT OF CN V

When testing CN V, ask the patient to close his or her eyes. Using a soft tissue, cotton, or paintbrush, lightly touch each of the three divisions of the trigeminal nerve (ophthalmic, maxillary, and mandibular), noting whether the patient detects stimulus.

MOTOR

The motor component of the fifth cranial nerve is tested by palpating the temporal and mandibular areas as the patient clenches and grinds the teeth.

CORNEAL REFLEX

The corneal reflex protects the cornea from drying out and from contact with foreign objects. The corneal reflex test (blink test) uses tactile stimulation of the cornea to examine the reflex pathway involving CN V for the sensory component and CN VII for the motor component.

Irritation of the cornea results in an eye blink. The test is elicited by using a wisp of cotton and gently touching the patient's cornea. This should result in a reflexive blink. In a practical setting, one has to ensure that the patient does not suffer a corneal abrasion from being a little too rough with this test or through repeating this test a number of times. It is of value to note that the same reflex can be elicited by squirting a little normal saline into the eye instead of using a wisp of cotton. An intact reflex response is consensual, involving automatic eyelid closure of both eyes.

HERPES

The trigeminal nucleus can harbor chronic herpes infections. After an acute infection, this ganglion may become the home of herpes as a chronic infection. When triggered, cold sores (mouth, herpes labialis) can break out, as can infections of the skin over any cranial nerve facial distribution—these breakouts can become severe and, when they involve the eye, become emergent. In such a case, steroids should *never* be used to treat the patient as it may result in permanent damage to the patient's sight or blindness.

TRIGEMINAL NEURALGIA

Trigeminal neuralgia is a painful spasm of the fifth cranial nerve, which may occur in one or more distributions of the trigeminal nerve, typically either V2 or V3. The pathophysiology is still poorly understood. The pain has a sharp stabbing quality lasting a few seconds, but may occur many times an hour when severe. Between the episodes there is no pain, although the patient may remain very fearful. The pain can both be triggered by an activity such as talking or eating, or it may just arise spontaneously.

■ CRANIAL NERVE VII: FACIAL NERVE

CN VII is involved in almost all movement of the face. In addition, it serves as a source of parasympathetic fibers to the submandibular and sublingual glands, increasing the flow of saliva from these glands. The parasympathetic innervation of the nasal mucosa and the lacrimal gland is also supplied by CN VII. It has a sensory component that carries information from the lateral border of the anterior two thirds of the tongue and the hard and soft palates. It is the moderator of the acoustic reflex, and forms the efferent limb of the corneal reflex along with CN V.

Signals for facial movement begin in the cerebral cortex. Upper motor neurons that project to the forehead do so bilaterally, but those upper motor neurons that project to the rest of the facial muscles do so only contralaterally. This results in bilateral innervation of the forehead muscles and contralateral innervation of the rest of the facial muscles. If there is a lesion of the upper motor neurons, such as a stroke, the patient will have a loss of lower face muscle function and intact forehead muscle function. Conversely, a lesion of the lower motor neurons, such as in Bell's palsy, results in a dysfunction of an entire side of the face.

The parasympathetic component of CN VII is important as it controls almost all of the major glands of the head. These glands are the submandibular, lacrimal, and sublingual glands, and mucous glands of the nose, paranasal sinuses, and hard and soft palates.

The sensory (afferent) components of the CN VII carry sensory information from the external auditory canal and taste sensation from the anterior two thirds of the tongue. The acoustic reflex moderates sound within the ear. In the ear, the sound travels from the tympanic membrane through the ossicles (malleus, incus, and stapes) to the fluid-filled cochlea, where it is detected by tiny hair cells, which in turn activate the primary auditory neurons to send signals to the brain. The stapedius muscle, which is innervated by CN VII, reflexively allows the stapes to be pulled away from the oval window into the cochlea, thereby reducing the intensity of the signal that reaches the cochlea and subsequently the volume of sound that is heard. This is a normal protective reflex arc that predominantly protects against high-frequency sounds; very low-frequency sounds are primarily transmitted through the bone to the ear.

A lesion in CN VII results in loss of innervation and, therefore, contraction of the stapedius muscle. This, in turn, results in failure of the acoustic (noise dampening) reflex. Patients with a lesion in CN VII present with hyperacusis.

TESTING CN VII

MUSCLES OF FACIAL EXPRESSION

Initially, inspect the face during conversation and at rest, noting any drooping or asymmetry of the face. Next, ask the patient to raise his or her eyebrows, frown, smile, and puff out his or her cheeks. You are looking for symmetry in motion indicating normal function of the facial muscles. Finally, ask the patient to squeeze his or her eyes shut tight and resist you while you attempt to pull them open. Once again, note asymmetry and weakness.

THE ACOUSTIC REFLEX

A patient may report hyperacusis, in which sounds seem louder than normal. To test this reflex, stand behind the patient and suddenly clap your hands behind one ear and then behind the other. Ask the patient if there was a difference in volume between the two.

THE CORNEAL REFLEX

The corneal reflex is described under Cranial Nerve V.

BELL'S PALSY

Bell's palsy is an idiopathic paralysis of the facial nerve. It can have a varied presentation, depending on where along CN VII the nerve is affected. The primary symptoms are acute onset of unilateral facial muscle weakness that involves the forehead as well as the lower parts of the face, impairment of taste, and hyperacusis. Involvement of the parasympathetic nerve fibers of CN VII can result in a reduction of secretory gland function. More than 80% of patients make a full recovery within 3 months. Upper motor neuron lesions may cause a facial palsy, but the clinical presentation differs from Bell's palsy in that there is no forehead involvement. In an upper motor neuron palsy, lower facial muscles on the side contralateral to the lesion lose voluntary control. The forehead muscles receive innervation from the ipsilateral hemisphere (as they are bilaterally enervated), thereby preserving their function (Figure 5.2).

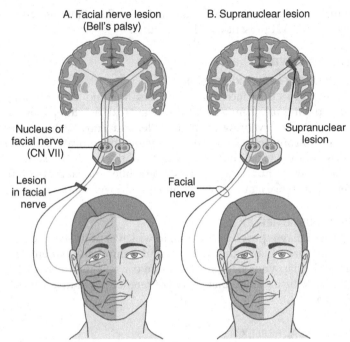

Figure 5.2 ■ Facial palsies: (A) lower motor neuron lesion in Bell's palsy with facial asymmetry and ipsilateral paralysis of upper and lower quadrants; (B) upper motor neuron lesion with facial asymmetry and loss of motor control in the contralateral lower quadrant only.

■ CRANIAL NERVE VIII: VESTIBULOCOCHLEAR NERVE

The vestibulocochlear nerve (CN VIII) transmits sound signals to the brain and provides a sense of position and movement.

Although referred to as the vestibulocochlear nerve, it is actually two distinct nerves: the vestibular nerve and the cochlear nerve. The vestibular nerve serves balance, and the cochlear nerve serves hearing. Peripherally, these two nerves run very close together, and therefore, although it is possible that only one of the two nerves is involved in a disease process, more often both are involved. Once the nerves enter the brainstem, their courses are more discrete and, therefore, less likely to be affected simultaneously. The sensory receptors of both components of this nerve are called hair cells.

TESTING CN VIII

AUDITORY SYSTEM

When assessing a patient's hearing, one can simply note "conversational hearing," but the sensitivity of this approach is only approximately 50%. Hearing can also be tested using the fingertips test, where the examiner rubs the fingers next to the patient's ear, first one side and then the other, and asks if the patient can hear it. Again this is not a very sensitive test.

More sensitive is the whispered voice test. The whispered voice test has at least 90% sensitivity and at least 80% specificity. Stand about 2 feet behind the patient to eliminate the possibility of the patient lip reading. Each ear is tested individually, beginning with the ear with better hearing. Block the ear not being tested. If necessary you can request that the patient use the finger to make a rubbing motion in the ear canal while blocking it to ensure masking the ear. Whisper as softly as possible a letter, a numeral, and another letter (e.g., "D, 3, S"). If the patient repeats the three items correctly, move on to the other side, using an unrelated letter–number–letter sequence. If the patient makes a mistake, whisper a new triplet to the same side. A patient fails this test if over two consecutive attempts there are more than three errors. For abnormal or questionable results, audiometric testing is warranted.

WEBER AND RINNE TESTS

Weber and Rinne tests are useful in distinguishing between conduction (sound waves are having trouble getting to the cochlea) and sensorineural (the problem is at the cochlea or beyond) deficits. A 512 Hz tuning fork is used for both the Weber and the Rinne tests.

The Weber test is for unilateral hearing loss. Strike the tuning fork lightly. Hold the vibrating fork firmly to the front of the skull at midline, and ask the patient if one side sounds louder than the other (Figure 5.3). If the good side seems to be louder, the damage is probably sensorineural. If the bad side seems to be louder, the damage is probably conductive. A patient with normal hearing will perceive the sound as roughly equal. This test assumes that the examiner knows ahead of time which side is hearing-defective and which side has normal hearing.

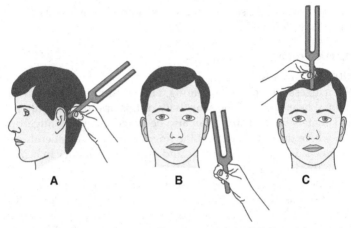

Figure 5.3 ■ Positions of the tuning fork during (A and B) Rinne's test and (C) Weber's test.

The Rinne test also tests for unilateral hearing loss, and it is generally performed in conjunction with the Weber test. It compares how he patient hears sounds transmitted by air conduction with those transmitted by bone conduction through the mastoid.

Strike the tuning fork, and hold the tuning fork lightly but firmly to the mastoid so that it is perpendicular to the ear. Ask the patient to tell you when the sound is no longer heard. Once the patient signals that he or she cannot hear it, quickly reposition the still vibrating tuning fork 1 inch from the auditory canal, this time holding the tuning fork parallel to the ear (Figure 5.3), and again ask the patient to tell you if he or she is able to hear the tuning fork. If the air conduction is louder than the initial bone conduction, this is a normal response and reported as a positive Rinne test. If bone conduction is definitely heard better than air conduction, this is strong support for conductive hearing loss, that is, something is inhibiting the passage of sound waves from the ear canal, through the middle ear apparatus, and into the cochlea. This is reported as a negative Rinne test. Note that in sensorineural loss, air conduction is still greater than bone conduction.

These are tests that need to be done in a quiet setting. Note that if the patient is suffering from profound unilateral deafness, the sound may still be heard through the opposite ear, leading to false test results.

VESTIBULAR SYSTEM

The vestibular system is involved in balance, body position, and orientation of the body with respect to gravity. Adjustments in body position and the body's ability to execute compensatory movements to maintain balance and position are a function of a number of reflex pathways.

UNILATERAL HEAD IMPULSE TEST

The unilateral head impulse test, also known as "head thrust test," tests the vestibulo-ocular reflex in a patient. It is a sensitive and specific test that detects a unilateral reduction in functioning of the peripheral vestibular system, generally caused by acute damage to the vestibular system. A functional vestibular system will identify any movement of the head position and allow for a rapid compensatory eye movement to ensure that the eyes remain fixated on their target.

Sit face to face with the patient, holding the patient's head from the front. Ask the patient to fix the gaze on a target in front of the patient (e.g., your nose) and turn the head very rapidly to one side while watching the eyes for presence or absence of any corrective movements. Repeat with the other side. When the head is turned toward the normal side, eyes continue to fixate on their visual target because the vestibulo-ocular reflex is intact for that side. When the head is turned toward an affected side, the vestibulo-ocular reflex fails, and the patient's eyes move with the head and then correct to refixate on the original target (Figure 5.4). This corrective movement is called a saccade. The presence of a saccade indicates vestibular as opposed to brainstem disease. The unilateral head impulse test should be used cautiously in patients with neck pathology because it involves rapid repositioning of the head.

CALORIC STIMULATION TEST

Caloric stimulation, like the unilateral head impulse test, relies on the vestibulo-ocular reflex. It is a test that uses temperature differences to diagnose damage to the vestibular component of CN VIII. Caloric testing of the vestibular nerve is seldom done during the bedside neurological exam, but may be done if vestibular nerve impairment is suspected. In this test, the head of the bed is placed at 30°. The eardrum should be examined before proceeding with this test to ensure that it is intact. Using cool water, irrigate the external auditory canal for 30 seconds. In a normal individual with

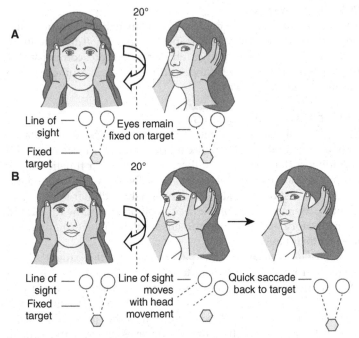

Figure 5.4 ■ Unilateral head impulse test.

an intact reflex, the eyes deviate to the irrigated side, followed by horizontal nystagmus to the contralateral side. The nystagmus appears after a latent period of 20 seconds and will persist for 1 to 2 minutes. After 5 minutes, the procedure is repeated, but this time using warm water. When warm water is used, the nystagmus is toward the irrigated ear.

The nystagmus seen in a normally functioning patient is an indication of a normally functioning cerebrum. In a comatose patient with cerebral damage, the fast phase of nystagmus will be absent. As a result, using cold water irrigation will result only in deviation of the eyes toward the ear being irrigated. Lack of nystagmus is an indication of brainstem dysfunction or death. The mnemonic COWS (cold opposite, warm, same) can help you remember these outcomes in a normal patient.

Cranial Nerves IX, X, XI, and XII

■ CRANIAL NERVES IX AND X: GLOSSOPHARYNGEAL AND VAGUS NERVES

TESTING THE GAG RESPONSE, SOFT PALATE ELEVATION, AND VOICE QUALITY

The glossopharyngeal (CN IX) and vagus (CN X) nerves travel their course very closely associated, which means that testing them independently is tricky; fortunately, it is also very seldom necessary. Damage to the glossopharyngeal and vagus nerves is rare, and this is best tested by eliciting the gag reflex. The gag response is easy to test, yet unpleasant for the patient, and consequently many providers will skip this in preference for symmetrical soft palate elevation and intact swallow. Intact swallow, however, does not indicate an intact gag.

SWALLOW AND PHONATION

Ask the patient to swallow. Is there any difficulty? Ask the patient to open his or her mouth wide and to say "ahh." The patient should be able to produce a clear sound, with the soft palate and uvula moving symmetrically. Changes in sound quality differ for central and peripheral lesions. There is a nasal, hoarse timbre to the voice with peripheral lesions, whereas central lesions produce a strained-sounding voice.

GAG

Gag is tested simply by poking the patient's uvula with a soft cotton swab or tongue depressor. As the name implies, a normal response is for the patient to gag. As this is an unpleasant test for the patient, most practitioners omit this unless there is evidence of a local lesion.

When the gag response is absent, it is generally quite obvious. Not only will you not see a reaction, but patients will state that the cotton swab did not bother them at all and will remain quite comfortable while you poke at their throats. The only way to incorrectly assess this test is to poke the patient's throat so hard in an attempt to get a response that you elicit a pain withdrawal response, prompting the patient to tell you he or she is uncomfortable.

Although testing the gag has a relatively low yield in general neurology, the lack of a gag response can be an important clinical finding. Where there is a strong need to rule out certain pathologies, testing the gag is required, and other tests should not be relied on. Lack of a gag may be due either to a sensory (afferent, CN IX) or a motor (efferent, CN X) conduction problem. Testing the soft palate for a symmetric raise (CN IX) in conjunction with the gag reflex may help narrow the etiology more closely. Although loss of gag can be a function of a serious underlying pathology, it should be remembered that approximately 20% of normal people have a minimal or absent response.

The lack of gag is present in a handful of cranial nerve pathologies, including cranial nerve tumors such as a glomus tumor (very rare) or a Chiari malformation (a little less rare).

■ CRANIAL NERVE XI: ACCESSORY NERVE

The accessory nerve (CN XI) is a purely motor nerve that innervates the sternocleidomastoid muscle and the upper fibers of the trapezius muscle. Damage to CN XI occurs in cases of neck injury, trauma, tumor, nerve lesion, or infarction. Damage to CN XI is rare.

TESTING THE TRAPEZIUS AND STERNOCLEIDOMASTOID MUSCLES

Testing the CN XI involves testing the trapezius and sternocleidomastoid muscles. Before testing motor function, observe the muscles for bulk. Wasting of one of these muscles may be an indication of lower motor neuron damage. Once bulk has been assessed, strength should be tested.

The trapezius muscle strength is tested using the shoulder shrug test. This is performed by asking the patient to shrug his or her shoulders against the manual resistance of your hands. Ensure that the patient is not using his or her arms to support the shoulders during this test.

Read rotation against resistance tests the sternocleidomastoid muscle contraction. To effect this test, the patient rotates the head laterally against manual resistance.

Lower motor neuron lesions produce weakness of both the trapezius sternocleidomastoid muscles on the same side. Upper motor neuron lesions produce sternocleidomastoid weakness on the same side as the lesion and contralateral trapezius weakness.

■ CRANIAL NERVE XII: HYPOGLOSSAL NERVE

The hypoglossal nerve is CN XII and controls movement of the tongue, which is key in speech, food manipulation, and swallowing. The hypoglossal nerve is seldom affected; however, the test is easy enough to include in the bedside neurological exam. Ask the patient to stick out his or her tongue; if there is a CN XII lesion, the patient's tongue will deviate to one side (Figure 6.1). If it is a lower

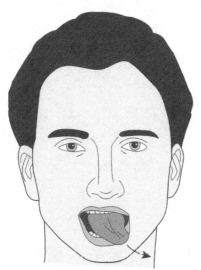

Figure 6.1 ■ Tongue deviation due to CN XII lesion.

motor neuron lesion, the protruded tongue will deviate toward the side of the lesion combined with the presence of fasciculations or atrophy. With an upper motor neuron lesion, the tongue will deviate away from the side of the lesion without fasciculations or atrophy.

Another way to test CN XII is by having the patient press the tongue against the inside of the cheek. You can then press this spot on the outside of the cheek and gauge how strongly the patient is able to resist you.

Testing Motor Strength

Weakness is a reduction in muscle strength and is a common complaint in primary care (see Chapter 17). Weakness may affect a few muscles or a large group of muscles. It may occur acutely or gradually.

Voluntary movement is initiated in the motor cortex at the posterior aspect of the frontal lobe. The signal is transmitted through the upper motor neurons, which synapse with the lower motor neurons in the anterior horn cells (or, in the case of the cranial nerves, in the motor nuclei). Lower motor neurons transmit impulses to the neuromuscular junction to initiate muscle contraction (Figure 7.1). Upper and lower motor dysfunction is discussed more completely under the section "Motor System Dysfunction" at the end of this chapter.

■ MUSCLE FUNCTION

Muscle function is assessed by evaluating three factors: trophic state, tone, and strength.

TROPHIC STATE

Assess the size, shape, and symmetry of a muscle. Muscle wasting is known as atrophy. Disuse of muscles, through inactivity such as prolonged illness or having a body part in a cast, can lead to a reduction in both the mass and the strength of the muscles. Unless severe, atrophy can be reversed with exercise. In such cases, the patient will benefit from a good physical therapy program.

Hypertrophy is the enlargement of a muscle group. Hypertrophy can occur naturally as a result of growth and exercise. This

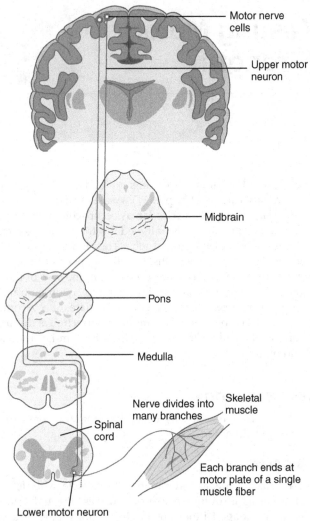

Figure 7.1 ■ Upper and lower motor neuron pathways.

is influenced by age, nutritional status, and natural hormone levels, especially testosterone, and is seen to occur at an increased rate during puberty in males. Hypertrophy can also be pathologic in diseases such as Duchenne's muscular dystrophy.

TONE

Muscle tone is the state of partial contraction of a muscle while at rest. Essentially, muscle tone is what makes muscles still feel somewhat firm while at rest and not intentionally being tensed. The muscle may be hypo- or hypertonic. Hypotonia is decreased muscle tone and may be seen in lower motor neuron lesions, spinal shock, and some cerebellar lesions. Hypertonia is increased muscle tone and manifests as spasticity or rigidity. Muscle tone is assessed by passive movement of a limb or of the particular muscle being assessed. Ask the patient to relax, and then passively move each one of the limbs, noting any resistance or rigidity that may be present. This is best done by comparing one side of the body to the other. When assessing for changes in muscle tone, there are some commonly used terms that are useful to know:

- **Clasp-knife phenomenon** is the resistance to passive movement with sudden give-way weakness toward the completion of the movement.
- **Paratonia** (gegenhalten) is the phenomenon of increasing rigidity through the passive movement being executed.
- **Cogwheeling** is stepwise increased tone through a particular passive movement.
- **Lead-pipe** resistance is uniform resistance to passive movement.

STRENGTH

Muscle strength is scored according to a standardized grading system from 0/5, when there is no voluntary movement, to 5/5, when there is movement against full resistance (Table 7.1). Have the patient pull and push against your resistance while isolating each muscle group. The muscle should be evaluated for strength and also compared with its contralateral part for symmetry.

■ PERIPHERAL MOTOR STRENGTH

A peripheral motor neuropathy is a result of a lesion(s) to the peripheral motor neurons. A mononeuropathy describes a condition in which only a single nerve or nerve group is damaged. A polyneuropathy describes damage to multiple nerves. The neuropathic lesion may be a result of an acute trauma or systemic illness.

Table 7.1 ■ GRADING SYSTEM FOR MUSCLE STRENGTH

5	Movement against full resistance
4	Movement against some resistance
3	Movement against gravity only
2	Movement with gravity eliminated
1	A flicker or trace of voluntary movement
0	No voluntary movement

Peripheral neuropathies do not pattern out into dermatomal or myotomal distributions, as you would see with nerve root damage and their associated radiculopathy, as discussed in the following.

In a peripheral neuropathy of systemic origin, such as diabetes, the nerves are affected distally in the extremities first. This is because longer nerves are affected more severely, and, therefore, changes predominate in the legs in a gradient from distal to proximal. Patients will have a triad of symptoms consisting of sensory loss in a glove and stocking distribution, weakness in the distal extremity muscles, and an absent Achilles reflex. Most distal polyneuropathies are purely sensory, or they affect the sensory and motor nerves together. Pure motor distal neuropathies are rare.

To assess for peripheral motor weakness, isolate the muscle groups being tested and assess them in a systematic fashion. It is useful to test the corresponding contralateral muscle immediately as a point of comparison.

■ **NERVE ROOT EVALUATION**

Radicular changes in strength (and sensation) stem from damage to the exiting nerve roots. When a nerve root is irritated or damaged, a specific pattern of muscle weakness will occur. This is because there is a set correlation between a particular group of muscles and a set of motor fibers that stem from a single nerve root. The pattern of weakness seen in nerve root compression is known as a myotomal distribution. Recognition of these patterns is helpful as it allows localization of the specific lesion (Tables 7.2 and 7.3).

Table 7.2 ■ CERVICAL NERVE ROOTS AND THE ASSOCIATED MYOTOMES

Most Important Nerve Root	Action	Predominant Muscle Group
C5	Arm abduction	Deltoid
C6	Elbow flexion	Biceps and brachioradialis
C7	Elbow extension	Triceps
	Finger extension	Extensor digitorum, extensor indicis, extensor digiti minimi
	Wrist flexion	Flexor carpi ulnaris
C8	Finger flexors	Flexor digitorum superficialis and flexor digitorum profundis
T1	Finger abduction	Interossei muscles

Testing muscle strength is best done by testing the left and right sides of the body simultaneously or in quick succession. This will allow the most sensitive evaluation of the

Table 7.3 ■ LUMBAR NERVE ROOTS AND THEIR ASSOCIATED MYOTOMES

Most Important Nerve Root	Action	Predominant Muscle Group
L1,2,3	Hip flexion	Iliopsoas
L2,3,4	Knee extension	Quadriceps
L4	Foot dorsiflexion	Anterior tibialis
L5	Great toe dorsiflexion	Extensor hallucis longus
S1	Hamstring	Knee flexion
S1, 2	Gastrocnemius	Foot plantar flexion

muscles being tested. All muscles are tested against resistance, be it against the examiner, or the patient's own body weight. In the upper extremities, it is preferable to test like-for-like, where the muscle being tested in the patient is pitted against the same muscle in the examiner. For example, use your bicep muscle to test the patient's bicep muscle. Because the patient's lower extremity muscles are so much stronger than the examiner's upper body muscles, where possible have the patient use his or her own body weight to test the muscles. For example, to test the dorsiflexion (anterior tibialis) of a patient, have the patient walk on his or her heels.

TESTING C5

The deltoid and bicep muscles are both innervated by the fifth cervical nerve (C5). The deltoid is innervated almost entirely by C5 and is very important as it is exclusively responsible for shoulder abduction past 30°. The bicep has both C5 and C6 innervation. C5 nerve roots are very sensitive to damage. Ask the patient to raise his or her elbows up past the 30° mark and then push up against your hands with the elbows while you offer resistance to this action (Figure 7.2).

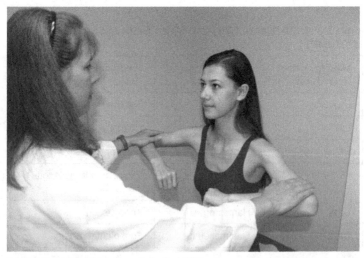

Figure 7.2 ■ Deltoid strength testing (C5).

TESTING C6

The bicep and wrist extensor muscles are both innervated by C5 and C6. Together with the brachioradialis, the bicep is involved in elbow flexion. Have the patient make fists with the arms bent in front of them and then pull inward against your resistance (Figure 7.3a). Wrist extensor testing is done by having the patient make a fist and extend the fist upwards and hold it there against resistance (Figure 7.3b)

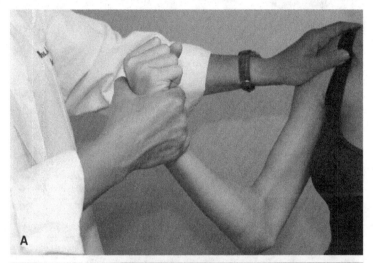

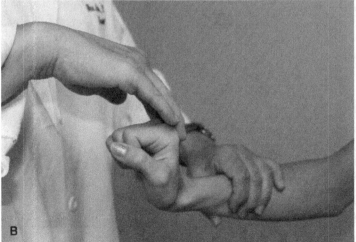

Figure 7.3 ■ Bicep (A) and wrist extensor (B) strength testing (C5/C6).

TESTING C7

The triceps, wrist extensors, and finger extensors are innervated by the C7 nerve root. The triceps extends the elbow. To test this muscle, have the patient begin from a position of flexion, extending out against resistance (Figure 7.4A). When testing a very weak

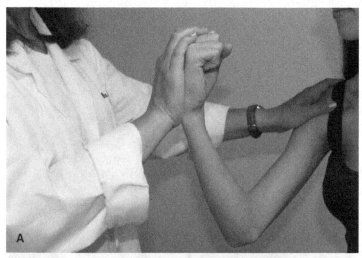

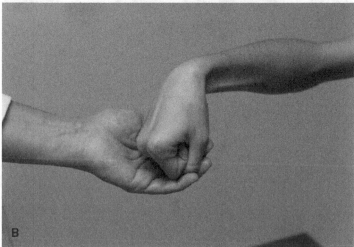

Figure 7.4 ■ Triceps (A) and wrist flexor (B) testing (C7).

triceps (grade 2), the patient may externally rotate the shoulder, whereupon momentum and gravity will allow the elbow to extend. Care must be taken to maintain the forearm in a horizontal position over the chest and to allow extension of the triceps horizontally to eliminate gravity. Wrist flexors are tested by having the patient make a fist and flex holding this position against resistance (Figure 7.4B).

TESTING C8

C8 is most easily tested by assessing finger flexion. Have the patient curl his or her fingers around yours or lock your fingers into the patient's flexed fingers, and try and pull them out of flexion (Figure 7.5).

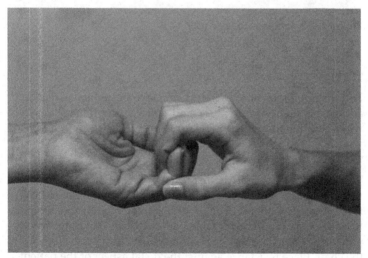

Figure 7.5 Finger flexors (C8).

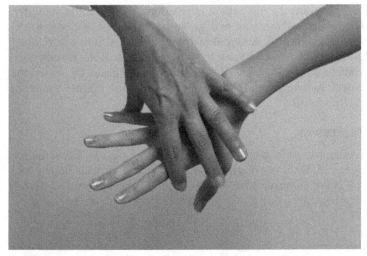

Figure 7.6 ■ Interossei muscles (C8/T1).

TESTING T1

Test the interossei muscles to test T1. Have the patient extend and adduct his or her fingers. Try and squeeze the fingers together while the patient resists you (Figure 7.6).

TESTING L1, 2, AND 3

The iliopsoas muscle is the main flexor for the hip and is innervated by L1, 2, and 3. To test this muscle, have the patient comfortably seated either on a chair with their feet barely touching the floor or on an examination table with their legs dangling. Ask the patient to then raise the knee straight up, lifting the thigh from the chair. Place resistance against the distal aspect of the patient's thigh (Figure 7.7).

TESTING L2, 3, AND 4

The quadriceps muscles are tested by having the patient sit on the edge of the examination table or on a chair with his or her feet off the floor. Stabilize the leg by placing one hand firmly on the

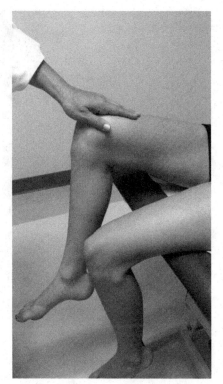

Figure 7.7 ■ Iliopsoas strength testing (L1, 2, 3).

patient's knee. The other hand is placed on the patient's shin to offer resistance to motion. Ask the patient to extend his or her knee against resistance (Figure 7.8).

TESTING L4

Heel walking is an important part of the strength exam. The anterior tibialis is one of the first muscles to weaken in many disease processes, for example, in multiple sclerosis. The patient who can heel walk bearing his or her own body weight has intact dorsiflexors. He or she also has good balance.

If a patient is too unstable to heel walk, you can test anterior tibialis strength by having the patient dorsiflex against resistance.

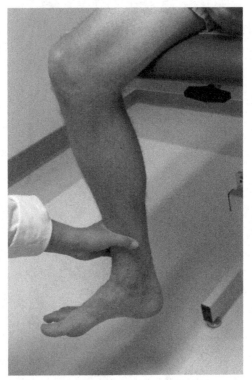

Figure 7.8 ■ Quadriceps strength testing (L2, 3, 4).

Testing for dorsiflexor strength is best done with the patient sitting in a chair or on an exam table. The patient's feet can either be hanging free or can be touching the floor. Ask the patient to dorsiflex; you can then place your hand over the dorsal aspect of each foot simultaneously and bear down (Figure 7.9). By having the patient stabilize his or her feet on the floor you will be able to use your body weight to test the strength of this strong muscle group.

TESTING L5

Extensor hallucis longus (EHL) muscle is innervated by the L5 nerve root. Ask the patient to raise his or her big toes against resistance to your thumbs. This should be done with both toes simultaneously for comparative purposes (Figure 7.10).

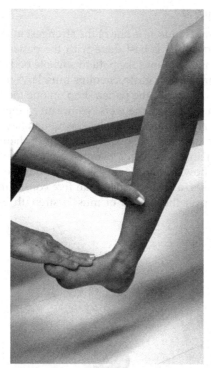

Figure 7.9 ■ Dorsifelxion of the foot testing anterior tibialis strength (L4).

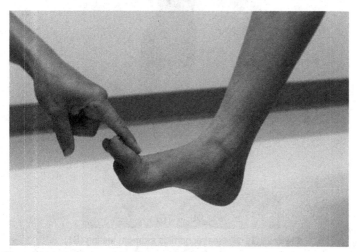

Figure 7.10 ■ Flexion of the big toe testing extensor hallicus longus strength (L5).

TESTING S1 AND S2

The gastrocnemius muscle is one of the strongest in the body. Testing the gastrocnemius is best done with the patient's own body weight. Toe walking allows the patient's whole body weight to be used as resistance to the gastrocnemius muscle. A more demanding test is to request that the patient hop on one foot and then on the other. Both of these maneuvers require an element of balance. For patients that have limited balance, you may have them face a wall and place their hands squarely in front of them on the wall for balance. Balanced in such a manner, ask them to rise up onto their toes and down again (Figure 7.11). In both the heel and toe walking exercises, a patient must take five consecutive steps (or toe raises) to meet the criteria of muscle strength being "within normal limits."

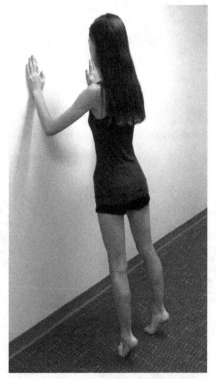

Figure 7.11 ■ Gastrocnemius strength testing (S1).

■ MYELOPATHY

A patient who presents with pain or changes in sensation along a particular dermatome may be managed nonoperatively. The presence of a myelopathy, however, changes the management strategy considerably, and then more urgent or emergent pathologies need to be ruled out, with cord or severe nerve root compression being the most important diagnosis to rule out. Put more simply, myelopathy happens late in the game, and there tends to be more at risk for the patient.

A lesion in the central nervous system may cause myelopathy. The most common cause of myelopathy is cervical spondylotic myelopathy (degenerative osteoarthritis), which is a result of degenerative processes in the cervical spine causing compression on the spinal cord and, generally, is a disease of age. Other causes include trauma, inflammation or infection (myelitis), or vascular disorder (vascular myelopathy). All may cause myelopathic symptoms.

The symptoms that a patient experiences are dependent on the location and extent of the lesion. They include symptoms such as paresthesias, weakness (including trouble lifting objects or dropping things), difficulty walking due to reduced balance, wide-based gait and decreased fine motor coordination seen in changes in handwriting, or difficulty buttoning clothes. In many cases, the onset of myelopathy is insidious, and the patient accommodates over time without realizing his or her deficiencies until they are quite severe.

On physical exam, the patient can be hyperreflexic and have pathologic reflexes such as positive Hoffman's or the presence of clonus (see Chapter 9, "Testing Reflexes," for further discussion on pathologic reflexes and how to test for them), diffuse weakness that is more pronounced in the upper extremities, or reduced sensation in his or her arms and hands. There may be atrophy of certain muscles if this has been a long-standing problem.

CERVICAL SPONDYLOTIC MYELOPATHY

Cervical spondylotic myelopathy is a condition that occurs typically in older patients. It is when the spondylosis (degenerative osteoarthritis) in their cervical spine progresses enough to cause narrowing of the spinal canal (stenosis) and impingement on the spinal cord. The cause of spondylosis may be due to inflammation, such as rheumatoid arthritis, degenerative discs, injury, or, less commonly, tumors, infections, or congenital abnormalities of the vertebrae. Cervical spondylotic myelopathy tends to be a progressive disease over years.

■ MOTOR SYSTEM DYSFUNCTION

Motor system dysfunction can result from damage or disease at any point along the motor pathway, either centrally and peripherally. Broadly speaking, the motor system is divided into two parts: the upper motor neuron system and the lower motor neuron system. Upper motor neurons originate in the motor cortex and project via the corticospinal tract to the anterior horn cells in the spinal cord. The upper motor neuron system is, therefore, defined at the neural pathway above the anterior horn cell of the spinal cord (Figure 7.1) or motor nuclei of the cranial nerves. Upper motor neuron disorders arise from lesions caused by stroke, tumors, and blunt trauma. Nerve fibers traveling from the anterior horn of the spinal cord or the cranial motor nuclei to the relevant muscles make up the lower motor neuron system. Common causes of lower motor neuron disease include trauma, infection, and autoimmune diseases.

Lesions in both the upper and the lower motor neurons can cause weakness. Different presenting symptoms result from damage at different levels in the motor system. The motor exam can give a good indication of where a lesion lies as upper and lower motor neuron lesions have very distinctive characteristics, as outlined in Table 7.4. When considering presenting symptoms, it is important to remember that an acute upper motor neuron lesion may initially present with a flaccid paralysis associated with both decreased tone and reflexes. As the lesion becomes less acute, an increase in tone and hyperreflexia usually develop.

Table 7.4 ■ **COMPARISON OF SYMPTOMS IN UPPER MOTOR NEURON AND LOWER MOTOR NEURON DISEASE**

Clinical Test	Lower Motor Neuron Weakness (LMN)	Upper Motor Neuron Weakness (UMN)
Weakness	Yes	Yes
Muscle tone	Decreased/flaccid	Increased/spastic
Muscle stretch reflexes	Decreased	Increased
Muscle atrophy	Profound	Minimal
Fasciculations	Present	Absent
Sensory disturbances	May have sensory disturbances	May have sensory disturbances

Testing Sensation   8

The evaluation of sensation is highly dependent on the willingness of the patient to cooperate during the exam. Sensation is a subjective test, and the results are what the patient says they are. Leading questions need to be avoided as they may cause the patient to modify his or her response. When testing a patient, differences in sensation that take more than a moment to discern are probably of no importance in the examination process.

When testing sensation, there are four basic skin sensations tested: light touch, pinprick, vibration, and temperature. Proprioception and then the higher order (cortical) aspects of sensation are also tested. The four skin sensations and proprioception each represent unique types of afferent receptors, and they travel in discrete pathways up the spinal column. Location and pattern of altered sensation can help localize the lesion. The loss of sensation may be peripheral (Table 8.1), such as a peripheral neuropathy from diabetes or carpal tunnel syndrome, or central in either the spinal cord or brain. When evaluating sensation, the site of the lesion may be deduced from the physical exam findings. For example, if the sensation maps out in a dermatomal pattern, then the nerve root level affected can be determined. Likewise, if the sensation is out completely from a particular point downward, then the level of a lesion in the spinal cord can be approximated, and complete lack of that sensation implies an upper motor neuron lesion, which gives a global defect.

■ DERMATOMAL SENSORY PATTERNS

Each pair of nerve roots that exits the spinal canal maps out a particular sensory pattern in a predictable fashion (Figure 8.1). The general pattern is similar in all people, although there is

Table 8.1 ■ COMMON PERIPHERAL SENSORY CHANGES

Type	Sensory Loss Location	Considerations	Examples
Distal peripheral neuropathy	From the toes upward to the feet and calves	This may be asymmetric, but will be a general altered sensation	Diabetes, multiple sclerosis, alcohol
Stocking-and-glove neuropathy	This is important to know as in most neuropathies, the distal portions (feet) lose sensation before the more proximal (hands)	The exceptions to the distal to proximal rule are metabolic neuropathies such as vitamin B_{12} deficiency	Metabolic disturbances, vitamin B_{12} deficiencies
Median nerve neuropathy	Thumb, index, and part of the middle finger of the affected side	The tinels test and the phalanges test, although commonly used in practice, have a very low sensitivity to diagnosis. Electromyography (EMG) is the gold standard for diagnosis	Carpal tunnel
Ulnar nerve neuropathy	4th and 5th fingers on the affected side	EMG is diagnostic	Cubital tunnel
Brachial plexus (or more distal nerve damage)	Entire arm from the point of pressure downward	This damage can be permanent or may take many months to heal	Brachial plexopathy, Saturday night palsy
Trigeminal neuralgia	CN V2 is the most common	Very difficult to treat medically. Surgical intervention is not a guarantee of symptom remission	
Significant pressure on the spinal cord or nerve roots in the spinal canal	Generalized decrease or loss of sensation—generally acute or subacute onset	This requires emergent MR imaging and specialty evaluation. Realize that it may cause irreversible damage and even death	Cauda equina syndrome

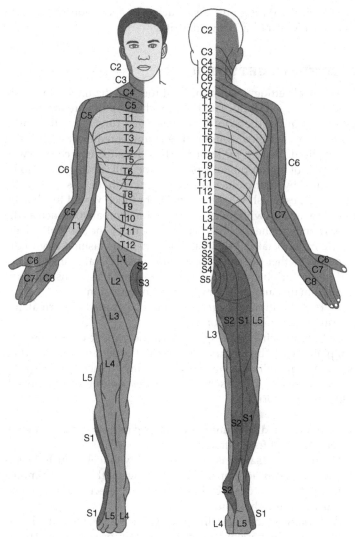

Figure 8.1 ■ Dermatomes.

some individual variation. Dermatomes apply only to nerve roots; sensory deficits from peripheral or central lesions will not follow dermatomal patterns. When evaluating sensation, move systematically through the distributions to allow yourself to form a clear understanding of any deficits.

■ TESTING LIGHT TOUCH

In a clinical setting, testing for light touch is the most commonly used test for sensation. The light touch receptors are located superficially under the skin. Touch sensation runs along the posterior tract of the spinal column. The stimulus required for this test is very light. Testing for light touch is done using a cotton swab or a wisp of cotton pulled from a cotton ball; testing can also be performed by lightly touching the patient with the tips of your fingers. First, establish what a normal light touch would feel like by touching an area with intact sensation for comparison, such as the face. Then with the patient's eyes closed, touch the areas of interest lightly from distal to proximal in a systematic fashion. Try to determine whether the loss of sensation is peripheral as in stocking-and-glove peripheral sensory loss or whether it patterns out more dermatomally such as in a nerve root compression.

The sensations they report should be graded as normal, hyperesthetic, hypoesthetic, or absent.

When testing with light touch, the patient often comes in complaining of "being numb." Have the patient explain what he or she means when using the word numb. When a patient describes change or loss of sensation, the descriptions commonly fall into three categories:

- **Pins-and-needles numbness** is classic paresthesias, or altered, sensation ("it feels different").
- **Decreased sensation** is a reduced ability to feel a touch. This is not necessarily accompanied by a change in the way a stimulus is felt. It can be described as though the affected area is being touched through plastic wrap.
- **Anesthetic skin** is literally areas where if a pin were stuck into that area, the patient would feel no pain or sensation. This is the same feeling as of not being able to feel one's skin after a lidocaine injection such as after going to the dentist.

Understanding loss of sensation is important not only in allowing a clinician to locate a lesion fairly quickly, but also in understanding other physical exam findings. For example, a decreased ability to feel is very important when considering a person's gait. When a patient cannot feel his or her feet, he or she will have trouble walking, which can, together with a loss of vibratory sense, lead to varying degrees of ataxia. A good example of this is seen in multiple sclerosis patients who develop glove and stocking hypoesthesias and consequently ataxic changes in gait.

■ PAIN (PINPRICK TEST)

Pain sensation runs along the lateral spinothalamic tract of the spinal column. As with temperature, loss of pain sensation can be a function of a peripheral neuropathy, a spinal cord lesion in the lateral aspect of the spinal cord, or a brain lesion in an area involved in integration of the sensory data.

Pinprick testing is done using a neurotip or unused safety pin. The patient should be able to make a clear distinction between dull and sharp sensation; allow the patient to experience both of these sensations on an unaffected area before testing begins. Have the patient close his or her eyes during the examination. You can switch between dull and sharp stimulus during testing and ask the patient to distinguish between those two sensations. Then with the patient's eyes closed, touch the areas of interest lightly from distal to proximal in a systematic fashion.

■ TEMPERATURE

Pain and temperature sensation both run along the lateral spinothalamic tract to the thalamus, where they synapse with higher order neurons. Temperature is tested either with vials of hot and cold water, or with something cool such as a metal tuning fork. Classically, the temperature should be 40°C to 45°C for hot and 5°C to 10°C for cold, as higher or lower temperatures can elicit pain responses rather than the desired change in temperature. In a clinical setting, a cool metal tuning fork is most commonly used. The patient is asked to describe the temperature: hot, cold, or no different. As pain and temperature fibers are closely associated, lesions of the spinothalamic pathways are generally found to affect both pain and temperature.

■ VIBRATION

Vibration sensation runs along the posterior aspect of the spinal column. As with proprioception, loss of vibration can be a function of a peripheral neuropathy, a spinal cord lesion in the posterior aspect of the spinal cord, or a brain lesion in an area involved in integration of the sensory data.

Vibration is tested by holding a tuning fork to the bony aspect of a patient's foot and then asking him or her to tell you when the vibration is no longer felt. As you are holding the tuning fork, you are able to compare how soon the patient loses a sense of vibration compared with when you lose the sense of vibration. This serves as a measure of how well the patient is able to detect vibration. A patient who is unable to feel more subtle vibratory sensations is said to have early extinction. A low-pitched tuning fork (pitch C 128) is a good choice for this test as it is easy to strike in a consistent fashion. Some of the more elaborate tuning forks have a numeric scale that allows for quantifying extinction time. Having such quantitative data can be useful when serial testing of vibratory sense over time is required and as a marker for disease progression. It is by no means necessary, and it is rarely used in the average bedside neurological examination.

■ PROPRIOCEPTION

Proprioception is the ability to perceive a sense of body position, analyze that information, and react appropriately (consciously or unconsciously) to the stimulation. Put simply, it is the ability to know where a body part is without having to look.

The ability to tell the position of one's body parts, known as joint position sense, is important in being able to function on a daily basis. Proprioception allows you to scratch your head without looking in the mirror or walk up a flight of stairs without having to see your feet or each stair. Loss of the ability to feel one's feet, and therefore not to know where one's toes are, affects balance, gait, and stability. The inability to tell where one's hand or arm is affects the smoothness of arm movement and the ability to be able to manipulate things in that hand.

Proprioceptive fibers run along the posterior column pathways of the spine. Loss of proprioception can be a function of a peripheral neuropathy, a spinal cord lesion in the posterior aspect of the spinal cord, or a brain lesion in an area involved in integrating proprioceptive information in the cerebellum, thalamus, and parietal lobes.

Clinically, joint position sense is measured with joint position matching tests that measure a patient's awareness of an externally imposed passive movement, or the ability to recreate a demonstrated position without the aid of vision.

One of the basic tests for proprioception is manipulation of the big toe. This is done by having the patient close his or her eyes. Move the toe upward, and tell the patient that is an upward movement. Similarly, move the toe downward, and tell the patient that this is down. Then randomly select a direction, and request the patient to identify in which direction you have now moved his or her toe (Figure 8.2). A repeat of three movements is usually sufficient to gain an understanding of the patient's ability to sense direction. With this test it is important to remember to hold the big toe on the sides and not the dorsal and plantar aspect of the toe, so as not to give the patient the advantage of being able to sense direction through changes in finger pressure as you move the toe.

The diseases that typically affect proprioception, such as multiple sclerosis, B12 deficiency, and peripheral neuropathy, tend to affect the lower extremities before the upper extremities, so, generally, it is enough to test only the lower extremities.

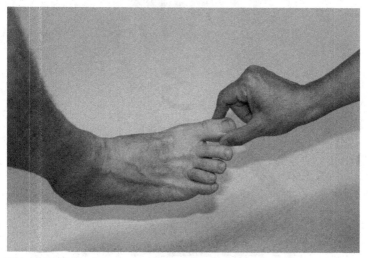

Figure 8.2 ■ Testing proprioception by manipulation of the big toe.

■ CORTICAL SENSATION (HIGHER ORDER SENSORY TESTING)

STEREOGNOSIA

Stereognosia is the ability to identify an item by feel. To test stereognosis, ask the patient to close his or her eyes and identify an object you place in the patient's hand. Use something that is recognizable such as a pen. Repeat this with the other hand using a different object. An inability to discern the object in this testing points strongly to either a dorsal column system lesion or a lesion in the sensory cortex of the parietal lobe.

GRAPHESTHESIA

Graphesthesia is the ability to discern what is being written on one's hand without seeing it. To test graphesthesia, ask the patient to close his or her eyes and identify a number or letter written on the palm of the patient's hand with a blunt object (Figure 8.3).

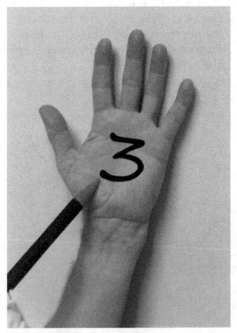

Figure 8.3 ■ Testing graphesthesia.

Repeat on the other hand with a different letter or number. Graphesthesia deficits are indicative of cortical damage.

EXTINCTION

Extinction is the ability to distinguish two different stimuli simultaneously. Have the patient close his or her eyes, and touch a part of the patient's body. The patient can then open his or her eyes and point to where he or she was touched. Have the patient close the eyes again, and for a second time touch the patient, but this time on two different sites that are on different sides of the body (e.g., left and right hand) (Figure 8.4). A normal result is that the patient can then tell you where he or she was touched. If the patient can point out only one of the two places, then extinction is present. The touch that is not felt is said to be extinguished. Extinction is seen with lesions of the sensory cortex in the parietal lobe. The extinguished sensation is on the side opposite to that of the damaged cortex.

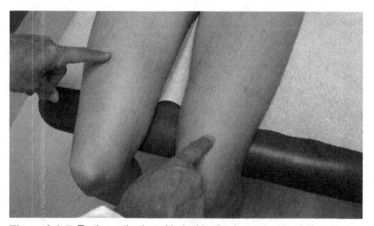

Figure 8.4 ■ Testing extinction with double simultaneous stimulation.

Testing Reflexes 9

Reflexes are a key component of a neurological exam. They are an objective test requiring little participation from the patient. There are many different reflexes, but for the purposes of this discussion we consider only the most commonly tested reflexes in a clinical setting (Table 9.1).

Table 9.1 ■ REFLEXES COMMONLY TESTED IN A NEUROLOGICAL EXAMINATION

Reflex Tested	Sensory and Motor Neurons Involved	Type of Reflex
Pupillary	CN II and III	Autonomic reflex
Corneal	CN V and VII	Superficial reflex
Gag	CN IX and X	Superficial reflex
Biceps	C5 and C6	Deep tendon reflex
Triceps	C6 and C7	Deep tendon reflex
Brachioradialis	C6, C7, and C8	Deep tendon reflex
Hoffman's	C6, C7, and C8	Deep tendon reflex
Patellar	L2, L3, and L4	Deep tendon reflex
Achilles	S1 and S2	Deep tendon reflex
Plantar	S1 and S2	Superficial reflex
Anal wink	S4 and S5	Superficial reflex

The basic structure of all reflexes is a sensorimotor arc, which involves a sensory signal and some kind of motor response. Monosynaptic reflexes (Figure 9.1A) are the most basic with direct synapse between the sensory fiber and the motor neuron. Polysynaptic reflexes may have several interneurons and synapses with varying complexity (Figure 9.1B).

A. A **monosynaptic reflex** has a single synapse between the afferent and efferent neurons.

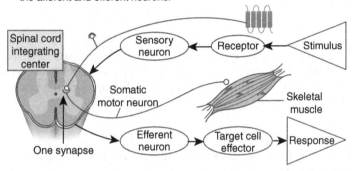

B. **Polysynaptic reflexes** have two or more synapses.

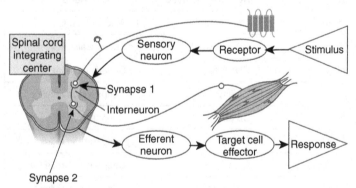

Figure 9.1 ■ Monosynaptic (A) and polysynaptic (B) reflex arcs.

■ DEEP TENDON REFLEXES

The deep tendon reflex, also known as stretch reflex or myotatic reflex, is a simple monosynaptic spinal reflex (Figure 9.2). The

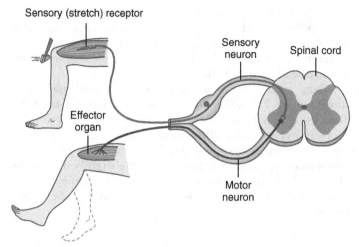

Figure 9.2 ■ A simple stretch reflex arc.

reflex is activated by stretching the tendon or a specific muscle, which can be done with a sharp tap from a reflex hammer. It is important to have the patient sit symmetrically and in a relaxed fashion for this testing. An isolated reduction in a reflex indicates a disruption of the reflex arc. This disruption may be at any point along the reflex pathway. For example, if a patient has had a total knee replacement the stretch receptors in the patellar ligament will be absent, disrupting the reflex arc resulting in an absent patellar reflex (areflexia).

Hyperreflexia (an excessive reflex response) may result from a disruption in the central nervous system reflex damping effect. When this damping is removed, there is nothing to moderate the reflex response, which results in hyperreflexia. Think of the disinhibition of the reflex arc, when due to pathology, as a top–down process: The lesion can affect everything below, or more caudal, to itself. Thus, a cervical lesion may affect the lower extremities but a lumbar lesion will never affect the upper extremities. For example, a cervical cord lesion may cause hyperreflexia in both upper and lower extremities. When a patient comes into clinic with a lumbar complaint, it is important to check his or her upper extremity reflexes as well as those in the lower extremities as the problem may not be (or may not exclusively be) in the lumbar area.

Hyporeflexia is common in large muscle-bound men and heavier patients. Certain drugs or medical conditions can also influence the reflex response, such as stimulants, hyperthyroidism, and serotonin syndrome. Marijuana causes quite marked hyperreflexia, due to the disinhibition of the reflex arc.

Deep tendon reflexes are graded in a semiquantitative manner where 0 is no sign of a reflex, 1+ shows a trace of a reflex, 2+ is a normal reflex, 3+ demonstrates hyperreflexia, and 4+ is hyperreflexia with clonus (Table 9.2). When testing reflexes, remember that people do not inherently all have the same reflex responses; a patient may have slightly augmented reflexes, which are symmetric and stable over time, or he or she may have little to no reflexes, which can both be normal variations.

Table 9.2 ■ REFLEX GRADING TABLE

Description	Grade
Mute	0
Hyporeflexic	1+
Normal (standardized patient)	2+
Hyperreflexic	3+
Hyperactive with clonus present	4+

BICEPS REFLEX

The biceps reflex is best tested by placing your thumb directly on the biceps brachii tendon (Figure 9.3). Using the reflex hammer, firmly strike your thumb and feel for the reflex response. The test activates the stretch receptors inside the biceps brachii and induces a reflex contraction of the biceps muscle resulting in a jerk of the forearm, which at times can be better felt than seen.

TRICEPS REFLEX

The triceps reflex is tested by directly tapping the triceps tendon with the reflex hammer while the arm is relaxed. This reflex can be

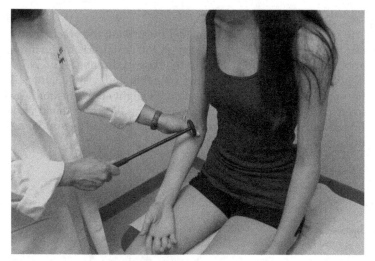

Figure 9.3 ■ Testing the biceps reflex.

tested either with the patient's arm at his or her side or with the patient's arm hanging loosely with the shoulder abducted and the forearm at 90° while you support his or her arm (Figure 9.4). You should observe a contraction on the triceps muscle.

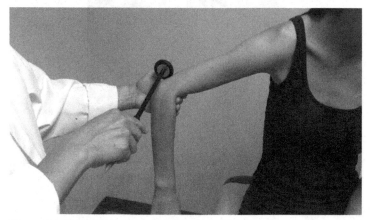

Figure 9.4 ■ Testing the triceps reflex.

BRACHIORADIALIS

The brachioradialis reflex is elicited by striking the brachioradialis tendon. The tendon is located on the radial side of the forearm, about 4 inches proximal to the base of thumb (Figure 9.5). A normal reflex response is the palpable and visible contraction of the brachioradialis muscle with slight elbow flexion. An inverted reflex response (abnormal) is the flexion of hand and fingers only. The brachioradialis reflex is recorded as normal or inverted.

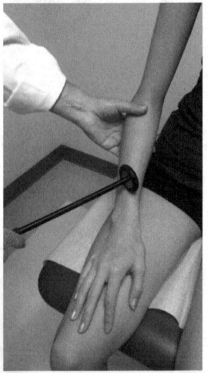

Figure 9.5 ■ Testing the brachioradialis reflex.

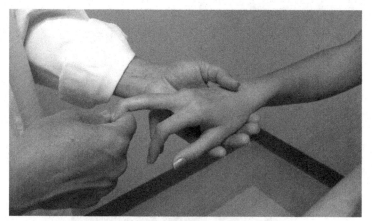

Figure 9.6 ■ Hoffman's reflex.

HOFFMAN'S REFLEX

The Hoffman's reflex, also known as the finger flexor reflex, is a deep tendon reflex that is normally completely inhibited by upper motor neurons. The test involves flicking the tip of the middle finger while gently supporting the wrist and palm of the hand. (Figure 9.6). A positive response is seen with flexion of the thumb and fingers. Unlike other deep tendon reflexes, it is graded as either present or absent.

PATELLAR REFLEX

The patellar reflex is elicited by striking the patellar tendon, which is located just below the kneecap (patella). A normal reflex is the sudden kicking (extension) of the lower leg (Figure 9.7).

ACHILLES REFLEX

The Achilles reflex is elicited by holding the patient's relaxed foot slightly in dorsiflexion with one hand and striking the Achilles tendon with the reflex hammer (Figure 9.8). A normal response is plantar flexion of the foot, which can be both seen and felt.

CLONUS

Clonus is the rapid, involuntary, rhythmic contraction of a muscle group after sudden muscle stretch. It is a symptom of spasticity,

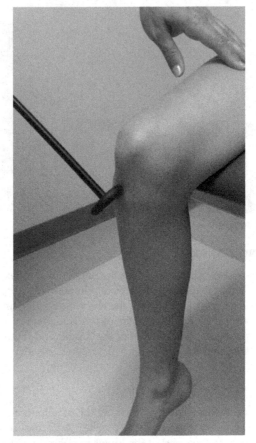

Figure 9.7 Testing the patellar reflex.

which occurs as a result of a lesion in the upper motor neurons. Most commonly, specific testing for clonus is done at the ankle, and as a result, ankle clonus has become synonymous with the term clonus. Although clonus is usually encountered in the ankle, it may be elicited in both the upper and the lower extremities.

Ankle clonus is tested by having the patient sit relaxed, with his or her feet dangling free. With one hand stabilizing the lower leg, use the other hand to dorsiflex the foot rapidly (Figure 9.9).

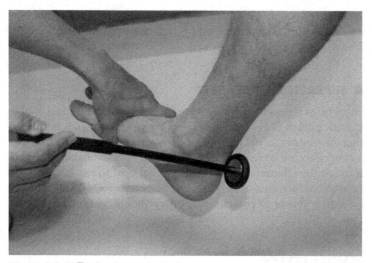

Figure 9.8 ■ Testing the Achilles reflex.

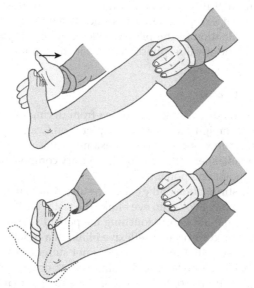

Figure 9.9 ■ Ankle clonus.

Absence of response is normal. Beating of the foot (rapid flexion and extension) is abnormal and is documented as 1 beat, 2 beats, 3 beats, or sustained clonus, which is more than 3 beats.

■ SUPERFICIAL REFLEXES

Superficial reflexes are motor responses to direct stimulation of a specific part of the body. These are polysynaptic reflexes requiring that the sensory signal must not only reach the spinal cord, but also ascend the cord to reach the brain. The signal then has to descend through the efferent neurons in the spinal cord to reach the motor neurons, which cause the observed response. Superficial reflexes are either absent or present. Symmetry should be noted as, when performing this test, significantly asymmetric results are abnormal.

PLANTAR REFLEX

The normal plantar response occurs when stimulation of the lateral aspect of the foot and then across the ball of the foot to the base of the big toe with a blunt instrument causes flexion of the big toe (Figure 9.10). Extension of the big toe with this test is always abnormal, except in newborns, and is known as the Babinski sign. The evaluation of the plantar reflex can be complicated by voluntary withdrawal responses to plantar stimulation.

CORNEAL REFLEX

The corneal reflex protects the cornea from drying out and from contact with foreign objects (see Chapter 5 on Cranial Nerve V). The corneal reflex test (blink test) examines the reflex pathway involving cranial nerve (CN) V for the sensory component and CN VII for the motor component.

Tactile stimulation of the cornea results in an irritating sensation that normally evokes an eye blink. The test is elicited by using a wisp of cotton and gently touching the patient's cornea (Figure 9.11). This should result in a reflexive blink. In a practical setting, one has to ensure that the patient does not suffer a corneal abrasion from being a little too rough with this test, or through repeating this test a number of times. It is of value to note that the same reflex can be elicited by squirting a little normal saline into the eye

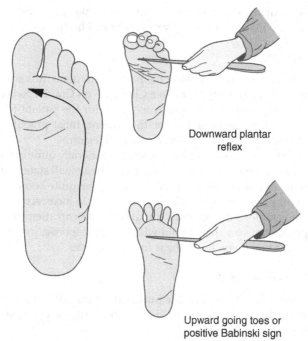

Downward plantar
reflex

Upward going toes or
positive Babinski sign

Figure 9.10 ■ Testing the plantar reflex.

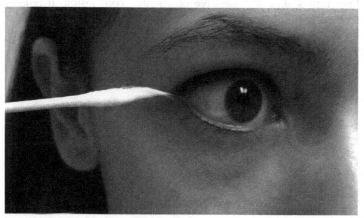

Figure 9.11 ■ Testing the corneal reflex.

instead of using a wisp of cotton. An intact reflex response is consensual, involving automatic eyelid closure of both eyes.

GAG REFLEX

Gag is tested simply by poking the patient's uvula with a soft cotton swab or tongue depressor (see Chapter 6 on Cranial Nerve X). As the name implies, a normal response is for the patient to gag. As this is an unpleasant test for the patient, most practitioners omit this unless there is evidence of a local lesion.

When the gag response is absent, it is generally quite obvious. Not only will you not see a reaction, but patients will state that the cotton swab did not bother them at all and be quite comfortable while you poke at their throats. The only way to incorrectly assess this test is to poke the patient's throat so hard in an attempt to get a response that you elicit a pain withdrawal response, prompting the patient to tell you he or she is uncomfortable.

ANAL WINK REFLEX

The anal wink reflex is a visible puckering at the edge of the external anal sphincter, which is elicited by touching the perianal skin with a pin.

LHERMITTE'S SIGN

Testing for Lhermitte's sign is done along with reflex testing. Lhermitte's sign is suggestive of a spinal cord lesion. It is performed with maximal head flexion by asking the patient to place his or her chin on his or her chest. The test is positive if this causes shooting, electric-like pain down the patient's front or back or in his or her lower extremities.

Balance and Gait 10

The evaluation of gait is a core component of a neurological examination. The ability to maintain a normal gait requires an integrated system of sensory input and motor coordination. Difficulty with gait—ataxia—may stem from either sensory or motor dysfunction.

The sensory component of gait involves balance. The underpinnings of balance include a functioning vestibular system (Figure 10.1), proprioception of the lower extremities, and sight. Two of these three things need to be present at any one time for the patient to maintain his or her balance and a normal gait.

The motor component of gait involves strength, coordination, muscle tone, and posture. These involve the upper and lower

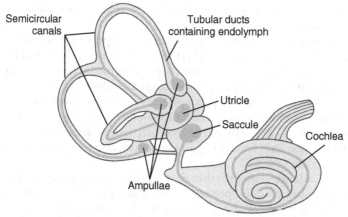

Figure 10.1 ■ The vestibular system: semicircular canals and otolith organs.

motor neurons, the cerebellum, and the extrapyramidal system. Disruption of the complex interaction of these factors leads to gait abnormalities. For further discussion on muscle strength and tone, please refer to Chapter 7.

■ EXAMINATION OF GAIT

The examination of gait begins as soon as the patient enters the examination room. To better judge gait, have the patient walk a timed fixed distance; this will allow comparisons over serial visits. Posture should be noted, as should any deformities. Gait is divided into two phases: the stance phase, where the foot is on the ground, and the swing phase, where the foot is moving forward. Most problems with gait are apparent in the stance phase as this is both the longest phase and the weight-bearing portion of the walk.

Observe the width of the gait. There should be 2 to 4 inches between the patient's heels as the patient walks. Patients widen their gait to improve balance and stability. Wider-based gaits can be indicative of pathologies such as vestibular dysfunction (Meniere disease, benign positional vertigo, middle ear viral infections), loss of proprioception or sensation due to a peripheral neuropathy, or unsteadiness due to a central lesion, in particular a cerebellar lesion. The development of a widened gait may also be a result of weakness in the lower extremities. Etiologies for this include nerve root entrapment, spinal lesion, and proximal muscle weakness.

The center of gravity in a patient lies approximately 2 inches in front of the second sacral vertebra (S2). Anteropulsion and retropulsion occur when the center of gravity is too far forward or too far behind, causing forward or backward acceleration.

The length of a step (amplitude) is the measurement from the heel of one foot to the heel of the other foot (Figure 10.2). In most patients, this is 14 to 16 inches. Step length decreases with increased age. Pain and other pathologies can also reduce the length of a person's step.

Cadence is the rhythm of a walk, or, more precisely put, the number of steps per unit time. Have the patient walk the passageway; there should be a smooth rhythm that measures roughly 100 steps per minute. Each person has a preferred cadence. Cadence does not change with aging.

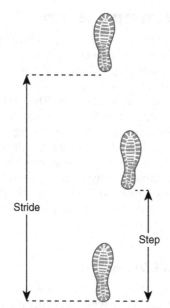

Figure 10.2 ■ Length of step and stride length.

Arm swing is a natural part of a walk, and fits the natural rhythm of the walk. While a large part of arm swinging is mechanically passive, movements are stabilized by active muscle control. Arm movement is important in overall gait stability. Lack of arm swing is typically seen in diseases that affect movement, such as Parkinson's.

Turning problems are common with any gait disorder; generally, turning is more difficult than walking. Make a point of observing how a patient negotiates a 180° turn. People without balance or gait problems usually can turn around in one or two steps. Blocked turns, and turns that require more than four steps, are typical of movement disorders such as Parkinson's, but can also be seen in frontal gait disorders[1] caused by cerebral or basal ganglia dysfunction. If a patient has less trouble turning than walking forward, a psychogenic disturbance is likely.

Note the patient's mechanics of walking: how high the feet are raised off the floor, circumduction of the legs, leg stiffness and degree of knee bending, difficulty with initiating or stopping gait, and any involuntary movements brought out by walking.

◼ PROVOCATIVE TESTING OF GAIT

Abnormalities in gait and balance may be brought out by asking the patient to do more difficult maneuvers.

To bring out subtle gait abnormalities or asymmetries, it may be appropriate in some cases to ask the patient to walk on his or her heels and then on the toes. The gastrocnemius muscle is one of the strongest muscles in the body. Gastrocnemius strength is most effectively tested by asking the patient to toe walk, thereby requiring that the patient lift his or her entire body weight. Heel walking allows assessment of the anterior tibialis muscle, which is a muscle innervated by the L4 nerve root. Foot drop is a result of damage to the anterior tibialis muscle and/or the L4 nerve, and is most readily picked up with heel-walk testing (see Chapter 7).

◼ EXAMINATION OF BALANCE

Tandem walking is a test of balance. This is done by asking the patient to walk a straight line while touching the heel of one foot to the toe of the other with each step (Figure 10.3). Patients with balance trouble, reduced sensation in their feet, or lack of proprioception will have particular difficulty with this task, since they tend to have wide-based and unsteady gaits, and become more unsteady when attempting to keep their feet close together. In a similar fashion, asking a patient to stand on one foot or hop on one foot will be challenging for the patient populace with balance difficulties.

The Romberg test utilizes vestibular function, proprioception of the lower extremities, and sight to deductively evaluate balance. Removal of sight (one of the three factors) will result in the patient's being required to use the other two for balance. This then allows us to determine that both of the remaining requirements are functional, as both would then be required for the patient to maintain balance. If the patient is unable to maintain his or her balance with eyes closed, but is able to do so with eyes open, then it may be concluded that either proprioceptive or vestibular function have been compromised. It should be noted that there are a few key parts to the Romberg test:

1. The patient should stand with feet close together to eliminate compensation from a wide-based gait (Figure 10.4). In some

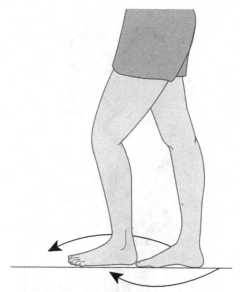

Figure 10.3 ■ Tandem walk.

populations, it is unreasonable to have the patient stand with feet touching—this is fine as long as the feet are close enough together to disallow for compensation.

2. The patient (with feet placed close together) needs to be able to stand balanced with eyes open. The inability to do this indicates a cerebellar lesion.

3. Do not allow the patient to fall as he or she closes the eyes!

■ GAIT AS A MEASURE OF FUNCTIONAL CAPACITY

When examining a patient's gait, one can also measure the patient's functional capacity, if need be. Functional exercise capacity tests are measurements of distance walked within a time frame or, conversely, the time that it takes to walk a set distance. In multiple sclerosis patients, one of the measures of disease progression is a 25-foot timed walk. Done at each office visit, this can show trends in functional exercise capacity. This is similar to the American Thoracic Society guidelines for a timed 6-minute walk test for

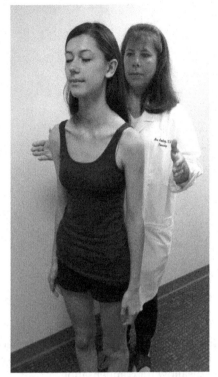

Figure 10.4 ■ Romberg test.

patients with severe cardiac or pulmonary disease as a measurement of response to medical intervention or a predictor of morbidity and mortality.

■ NAMING NEUROLOGIC GAITS

The antalgic gait is seen in patients who avoid certain movements to evade acute pain. The compensatory maneuvers used by patients are an attempt to achieve reduced weight-bearing time on the painful limb, avoidance of impact loads, reduced joint excursion, and minimization of activity in muscles that cross the joint. The person's body weight is transferred away from the side that hurts, lengthening the time spent on the uninjured side. This results in an arrhythmic gait with decreased swing in the good leg, creating a shorter step length on the uninvolved side, decreased walking speed, decreased cadence, and the absence of forceful foot contact or push-off.

If a painful hip is causing the problem, the patient also shifts his or her body weight over the painful hip, decreasing the pull of the abductor muscles, which decreases the pressure on the femoral head from more than two times the body weight to approximately body weight. This gait would be seen in acute trauma, for example when a patient stubs a toe or twists an ankle.

The Trendelenburg gait or myopathic gait is caused by weakness of the hip abductors. When the hip abductor muscles (gluteus medius and minimus) are weak, the stabilizing effect of these muscles during gait is lost. This condition makes it difficult to support the body's weight on the affected side. When there is an abductor weakness, the pelvis drops on the contralateral side because the ipsilateral hip abductors do not stabilize the pelvis to prevent the droop when unsupported. The patient will therefore compensate by swinging his or her body over the affected hip to place the center of gravity over the hip, thereby reducing the degree of the pelvic drop (Figure 10.5). A Trendelenburg gait is commonly seen in the muscular dystrophies or in poliomyelitis.

The hemiplegic gait is a result of weakness to one side of the body. When walking, the patient will hold his or her arm to one side, flexed and adducted owing to hypertonicity of the flexor muscles in the upper extremities. There will be loss of normal arm swing. The foot on the affected side will circumduct due to foot drop and extensor hypertonia in the lower limb (Figure 10.6). This is most commonly seen in stroke.

Spastic gait has a stiff, foot-dragging quality of walk caused by a long muscle contraction on one side (Figure 10.7). This gait may be seen with many brain and spine lesions, such as brain tumors, multiple sclerosis, brain trauma, and cerebral palsy. It may also be seen in the patient with liver failure and pernicious anemia.

Steppage gait or neuropathic gait is due to the patient trying to lift his or her leg high enough during walking so that the toe does not catch or the foot does not drag on the floor (Figure 10.8). This is seen in patients with weakness of dorsiflexion (anterior tibialis muscle) that causes foot drop. Common causes of this gait, if unilateral, include peroneal nerve palsy and L4 myelopathy. If

The Trendelenburg Test

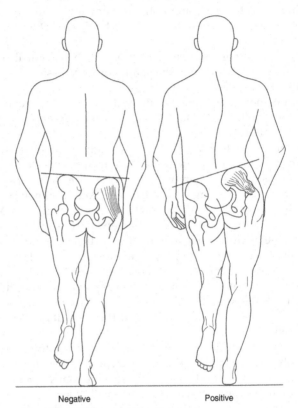

Negative   Positive

Figure 10.5 ■ Trendelenburg gait.

bilateral, causes include amyotrophic lateral sclerosis, the dystrophies, and other peripheral neuropathies, including those associated with uncontrolled diabetes.

A hypokinetic gait seen in parkinsonian patients has an overall slowness of movement, with a reduction of the step amplitude but an unchanged or slightly increased cadence (Figure 10.9). In addition to reduced stride length and walking speed during free ambulation, and changes in cadence rate, turning is *en bloc* like a statue.

Festination is another typical and unique gait pattern observed in Parkinson's disease. A festinating gait is a series

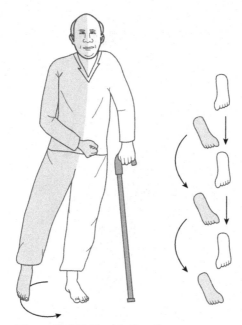

Figure 10.6 ■ Hemiplegic gait.

of rapid small steps done in an attempt to keep the center of gravity in between the feet while the trunk is leaning forward involuntarily.

Freezing of gait (FOG) is commonly seen in Parkinson's patients, although it is not specific to Parkinson's disease. Often, these patients have difficulty initiating movement and may also have difficulty stopping after starting. FOG is an interruption of gait that typically lasts a few seconds and is described by patients as a sensation of being glued to the ground, resulting in their inability to move despite making their best effort. FOG often has triggers such as clearance of an obstacle or narrow passage or unexpected sounds or visual stimuli. Conversely, certain visual and auditory stimuli, such as markings on the ground or rhythmic sounds, may aid in overcoming FOG. Fatigue, stressful situations, cognitive load anxiety, and depression may also elicit FOG, which is not specific to Parkinson's. It may also be seen with basal ganglia disease; with degenerative

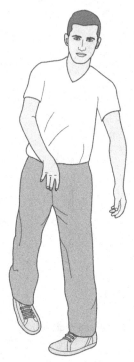

Figure 10.7 ■ Spastic gait.

disorders such as progressive supranuclear palsy, multisystem atrophy, or dementia; with Lewy bodies and in focal lesions of various brain structures; or with certain drugs such as haloperidol (Haldol).

The ataxic gait (ataxia) is characterized by the incoordination of voluntary movements. This presents as a broad-based gait that has a lurching quality, difficulty with turning, and difficulty walking in a straight line. The ataxic gait may be divided into two broad categories based on underlying pathology: cerebellar ataxia and sensory ataxia.

■ Cerebellar ataxia results from the lack of voluntary coordination of muscle movements that result from dysfunction of the cerebellum. The cerebellum is responsible for smoothly coordinating movement by integrating a significant amount of neural

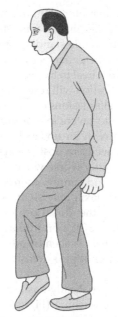

Figure 10.8 ■ Steppage gait.

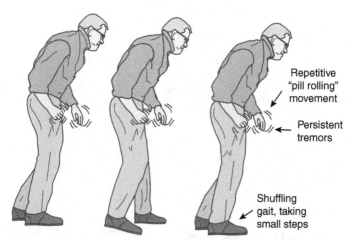

Repetitive
"pill rolling"
movement

Persistent
tremors

Shuffling
gait, taking
small steps

Figure 10.9 ■ Parkinsonian gait depicting small shuffling steps, forward tilt of trunk, and reduced arm swing.

information involved in motor planning and function. This gait is wide-based and uncoordinated, with staggering movements and truncal instability. While standing still, the patient's body may sway even while the patient's eyes are open. Patients will not be able to walk from heel to toe or in a straight line. The gait of acute alcohol intoxication will resemble the gait of cerebellar disease. Not all cerebellar lestons cause ataxia.

■ Sensory ataxia is due to severe loss of proprioception. Sensory ataxia presents itself with an unsteady "stomping" gait with heavy heel strikes, as well as a postural instability. These symptoms become significantly worse when the patient is asked to close his or her eyes and cannot, therefore, compensate with visual input. Sensory ataxia may stem from severe peripheral neuropathy, damage to the dorsal columns of the spinal cord, or dysfunction of areas of the brain that are important in positional information. This is seen in advanced neuropathy, as found in diabetes and multiple sclerosis.

Scissors gait characteristically has legs flexed slightly at the hips and knees such as crouching (Figure 10.10). A person with

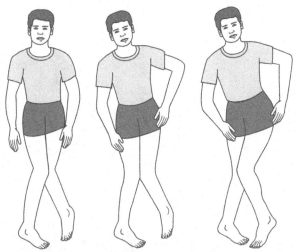

Figure 10.10 ■ Scissors gait.

scissors gait may walk with his or her knees or legs crossing or hitting each other in a scissorslike movement.

▨ **NOTE**

1. Frontal gait disorder is a broad term that describes a combination of findings, namely variable broadening of base, short shuffling steps, start and turn hesitation, moderate disequilibrium, preserved arm swing, and upright posture.

Testing Coordination

Classic texts describe coordination testing as a window into cerebellar function. This is true; however, when testing at the bedside it is important to remember that balance (vestibular system), vision, orientation (proprioception), and executive function (sequence processing) all contribute to the clinical impression of coordination. A patient with a tremor or with proximal muscle weakness may look uncoordinated. Alcohol, drugs, and certain medications may also influence coordination testing. The results of coordination testing need to be interpreted contextually with the greater medical picture including medications and patient circumstance in order to produce a meaningful assessment. Therefore, as straightforward as these tests are, they can be tricky to integrate into the final clinical assessment.

■ TESTS USED

There are a number of tests that may be used to evaluate a patient's coordination (Table 11.1). The finger-to-nose test is aimed at evaluating upper extremity coordination. Ask the patient to touch his or her nose with the index finger and then touch your finger that is placed in front of them (Figure 11.1). This is a basic coordination test that is easily executed even in those with limited cognitive abilities, as it requires only a single-step command and limited attention.

The finger-to-nose-to-finger is an elaboration of the basic finger-to-nose test already described. In this test, however, the patient is asked to touch his or her nose repeatedly with the index finger and then your finger while you move your finger to different locations in front of him or her. The patient should do this as

Table 11.1 ■ **COORDINATION TESTS**

Test Name	Test Is Aimed at
Finger-to-nose	Basic coordination test. Easily executed.
Finger-to-nose-to-finger	Allows extended observation time and reduces possible compensation by higher function processing.
Rapid alternating hand movements	Detecting loss of fine motor coordination. Good for high-functioning patients.
Heel-to-shin	Lower extremity ataxia. Accuracy is important, not speed.
Rapid simultaneous toe-tapping	Detecting loss of fine motor coordination. Good for high-functioning patients who may compensate using higher functioning processes.
Gait	Can be evaluated unobserved but requires the patient to be physically mobile.

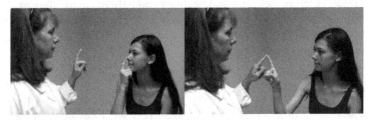

Figure 11.1 ■ Finger-to-nose coordination testing.

rapidly as possible. The advantage of this test is that it allows the examiner multiple visualizations of a rapid process and also serves to eliminate some of the compensatory cognitive processes exhibited by higher functioning patients.

The hand-slap test (or rapid alternating hand movement test) is a good test of coordination that can elicit some of the more subtle changes from baseline. In this test, patients are asked to tap their hands on their laps, rapidly alternating between the dorsal and palmar aspects of their hands (Figure 11.2). This test has the advantage of overcoming possible compensation in a

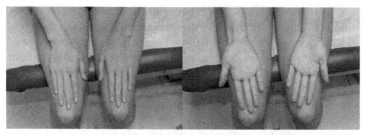

Figure 11.2 ■ The hand-slap test (or rapid alternating hand movement test).

high-functioning patient owing to its speed and its demand for simultaneous processing of the movement of both left and right hands.

Lower extremity coordination testing typically is heel-to-shin testing. In this test, the patient is asked to touch the knee with the heel of the other foot, and then run the heel down the length of the shin (Figure 11.3). This test is relatively easily executed, although it does require the heel to be traced exactly from the top of the kneecap down the full length of the shin, which takes a measure of understanding and physical flexibility. Speed is not important in this test, but accuracy is.

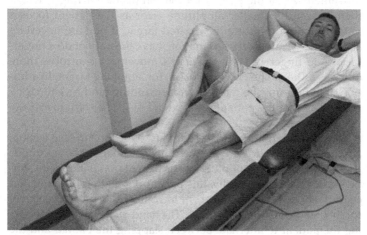

Figure 11.3 ■ Heel-to-shin coordination testing.

Foot tapping is the lower extremity equivalent of alternating hand movements. In this test, the patient is asked to tap their feet on the floor as quickly as possible. This test has the advantage of overcoming possible compensation in a high-functioning patient owing to its speed and its demand for simultaneous processing of the left and right feet.

The loss of ability to perform rapid alternating movements is called dysdiadochokinesia. Complete lack of ability to perform rapid alternating movement is call adiadochokinesia.

■ TESTING THE PATIENT

Speed is an important factor in these tests as it unmasks ataxic movements; however, in and of itself, it is a nonspecific finding. To detect mild cerebellar problems, the tasks should be more demanding.

In the finger-to-nose testing, simply missing the nose or being tremulous from finger to nose does not translate into un-coordinated movements. Look for a smoothness of movement versus the choppy lack of control seen in an attempt at move-ment and then overcompensation for the movement. Ataxia is the gross weaving (zigzag) of a finger that is poorly controlled as it moves deliberately between two points (Figure 11.4). Typi-cally, there is a large amplitude control problem on initiation of movement when the patient focuses on his or her finger, which then becomes a smaller amplitude error as the patient focuses more intently on hitting the desired target. If you are uncertain about what you see on examination, have the patient do a finger-to-nose-to-finger test—the patient's movement control is more obvious as he or she now has to aim for a moving target. In addi-tion, that task may be made more demanding (and revealing) by requesting that the patient fully extend his or her arm to execute the maneuver.

Rapid alternating movement tests, such as hand-slap testing, are more sensitive to early changes in coordination. For example, this is useful in the multiple sclerosis patient population with sub-tle ataxic changes; typically, this patient population is young and cognitively intact, allowing them to compensate more effectively for their coordination difficulties. The hand-slap test is simply ask-ing the patient to alternate between slapping the palmar and the

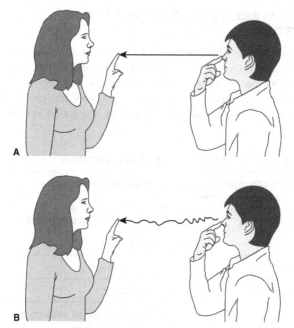

Figure 11.4 ■ (A) Normal finger-to-nose test and (B) abnormal ataxic movements.

dorsal aspects of the hand on his or her thigh. The key is to have the patient execute these movements of both hands simultaneously and rapidly so that there is no time to overthink about what is being asked of him or her.[1]

Lower extremity coordination is tested by heel-to-shin testing or rapid foot tapping. Heel-to-shin testing is executed by requiring that the patient draw a line with one heel along the other shin. Each side is tested. This test is not a function of speed but rather a function of precision. In an older or ill population, the ability to be flexible enough to execute this test is variable. It also requires more patient cognition than the finger-to-nose test.

Rapid toe-tapping is a fine coordination test in those patients who are unable to walk, not very flexible, or are so high functioning or low functioning that a test with not more than one command is needed. This test is an evaluation of rate and rhythm.

■ INTERPRETATION OF COORDINATION TESTING

In any of the coordination tests, slowness is a nonspecific finding. An irregular rate or rhythm of movement and difficulty making rapid movements aimed at a specific target are suggestive of cerebellar hemispheric lesions. Gait ataxia is more indicative of midline cerebellar involvement. In either case, the tested ataxia will be

Table 11.2 ■ ETIOLOGIES OF ATAXIA-LIKE FINDINGS

Possible Etiologies of Ataxia-Like Movements	Additional Confirmatory Test
Cerebella lesion	Swaying with eyes open and closed *
	Imaging
Paresis	Motor testing**
Proprioception	Big-toe test
Parkinson's	Associated classic pathognomonic symptom quadrad
Stroke or other supratentorial lesions	Imaging
	History
Alcohol or recreational drug use	Patient history
Medications	Patient history
	Known medication list
Tremor	Consistency (evenness) of movement during testing
	Known medical history
Vision abnormality	Known medical history
	Bedside vision testing (Snellen chart)

*This is a negative Romberg test, which, by definition, is positive if the patient is stable with feet well approximated and facing the examiner, and then starts to sway considerably or to fall over when the patient closes the eyes. At this point, it is good form to catch the patient. A small sway is not considered positive.

**Pay attention to the proximal musculature.

associated with a negative Romberg test. See Chapter 10 on balance and gait for a broader discussion on this concept.

Incoordination suggests a cerebellar lesion when excluding other influencing factors. When evaluating a patient with ataxic findings, first rule out the obvious complicating factors (medications, substance abuse, tremor). Rule out may be done rapidly, but should be approached systematically. Table 11.2 outlines some possible etiologies of ataxic-like findings and additional confirmatory testing that may be done.

■ **NOTE**

1. Do not confuse this testing with sequencing tasks such as the hand movement sequencing test, where the goal of the patient repeating a series of sequential hand movements is to evaluate frontal lobe functionality.

Imaging and EMG Studies

12

Plain films, computed tomography (CT) imaging, and magnetic resonance imaging (MRI) with their variations are the mainstays of neurological imaging. Each imaging modality has its advantages and careful consideration should be given to study choice. In this chapter, we will review the three most common imaging modalities used in neurology. As a general guide, Table 12.1 outlines the preferred imaging techniques for common neurological pathologies.

Table 12.1 ■ PREFERRED IMAGING FOR COMMON PATHOLOGIES

Tumor	MR
Demyelinating disease	MR
Infarcts—acute	MR
Infarcts—subacute/chronic	MR or CT
Acute hemorrhage	CT
Subacute/chronic hemorrhage	MR
Aneurysm	MR or CT
Skull fracture	CT
Degenerative spinal changes (spondylosis)	CT
Degenerative disc disease with or without radiculopathy or myelopathy	MR
Epidural abscess	MR
Spine fracture	CT

■ PLAIN FILMS

Plain x-ray films are an imaging modality where electromagnetic radiation is used to send particles through the body. Different parts of the body will absorb varying amounts of radiation based on their density, resulting in different amounts of x-rays passing through and exiting the body. The images are recorded on a computer or film that is sensitive to this radiation. Dense material appears white (hyperintense) on x-ray. The least dense material, such as air, is black on x-ray (hypointense). Plain films show a two-dimensional representation of the bony structures (Figure 12.1).

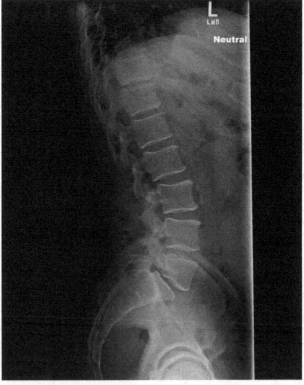

Figure 12.1 ■ Plain film of the lumbar spine shows a 2-dimensional representation of the bony structures.

Plain films are a valuable tool as they are quick and easy to take and affordable in comparison with other imaging choices. Before CT and MRI became routine diagnostic procedures, plain films were the mainstay of imaging in neurology. CT and MRI give much greater detail, but plain films are still useful in such cases as looking for spine instability with flexion–extension films and assessing degenerative changes and deformities of the spine.

Fluoroscopy is a form of x-ray. A specific area is focused on and low-dose radiation is pulsed or produced continuously to provide imaging of that body area in motion. Fluoroscopy is commonly used intraoperatively in spine surgery, where is it used in the establishment of location and in the guidance for hardware placement, and for needle guidance during steroid injections into the neck, spine, and sacroiliac joints.

■ COMPUTED TOMOGRAPHY SCANS

As with plain films, CT imaging is based on the variable absorption of x-rays by different tissues. It provides a form of imaging known as cross-sectional imaging. A motorized table moves the patient through a circular opening in the CT scanner. As the patient passes through the CT scanner, a source of x-rays rotates around the inside of the circular opening. Many different angles are collected during one complete rotation. This imaging is very rapid. A single rotation takes about 1 second. Multiple detectors record the x-rays exiting the section of the patient's body being irradiated. The information from the detectors is then sent to a computer for reconstruction of the image. The data from one rotation are compiled into one "slice" of a CT image. The primary plane of scanning is axial. The computer uses the axial images to reconstruct views in different planes, which is known as image reformatting. CT is excellent for evaluation of cortical bone, making it an excellent choice for detecting fractures of the spine (Figure 12.2). It can also be helpful for differentiation among fat, fluid, soft tissue, bone, and air.

CT imaging is not risk free. One of the greatest concerns is radiation exposure, especially if a patient has had numerous CT scans in the past. The use of iodinated contrast dye in a person who is allergic to iodine or who has poor renal clearance adds another level of risk. Having a history of contrast allergy is not

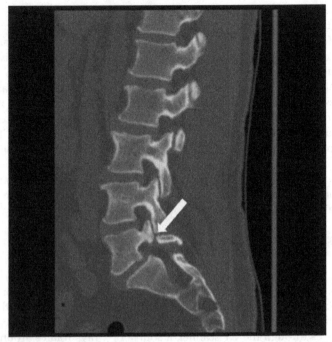

Figure 12.2 ■ CT image of the lumbar spine showing a pars defect at L5.

an absolute contraindication as there are now nonionic iodine agents available. If a patient's reaction is minor, the patient may be premedicated with steroids and Benadryl. Where a patient has poor renal function, iodine should be used cautiously and with liberal administration of intravenous fluids. Metformin is an oral hypoglycemic agent that is predominantly eliminated by renal excretion. Patients on metformin may take metformin until the day of imaging. Creatinine levels need to be drawn prior to CT imaging and 48 hours after injection of the dye before metformin is resumed. Patients may feel a warm flooding sensation as the dye is injected into the bloodstream, and they may experience a slight metallic taste.

Dense bone, metal, and patient motion can all create artifact in the CT imaging series. Imaging of the posterior fossa by CT is not ideal in view of the dense nature of the skull bone in this region making the imaging difficult to evaluate. Metal from dental fillings and surgical clips can interfere with the image. Patient size may also limit high-quality imaging, as it does with plain films. Pregnancy is an absolute contraindication to CT imaging.

A CT myelogram combines the use of a contrast substance with CT imaging. This is an invasive technique. A myelogram differs from a regular CT with contrast because in a CT myelogram, the contrast is injected into the subarachnoid space within the spinal column before the procedure. The dye then outlines the spinal structures, such as nerve roots and spinal cord, and allows the target tissue to be visible. A CT myelogram is useful in patients with extensive instrumentation in their spine, as metal-induced artifact in conventional MRI would obscure much of the structures being examined. Patients with non–MRI compatible implants, such as cochlear implants or pacemakers, are also good candidates for a CT myelogram.

CT angiography is used to detect blockages in the arteries or veins. It combines CT imaging with the administration of a contrast dye injected peripherally. The degree of narrowing or obstruction of a blood vessel can be seen on an angiogram of the brain, head, or neck. It is the gold standard in the evaluation of vascular disease of the brain and spine, including aneurysms, arteriovenous malformations (AVM), and vasculitis.

■ MAGNETIC RESONANCE IMAGING

MRI first came into its own as an imaging technique in the 1980s, although it had been the interest of some researchers since 1950.

MRI is based on exciting nuclear spin states with a radiofrequency generator in a strong magnetic field and measuring the induced current in receiver coils. MRI requires a strong, uniform magnetic field, which is known as its field strength. The field strength of an MRI magnet is measured in tesla (T). The stronger the magnet (MRI field strength), the greater the resolution of image. Although most clinical MRI machines operate at 1.5 T to 3 T, MRI systems are commercially available between 0.2 T and 7 T. The lower field strengths can be achieved with permanent magnets, which are often used in "open" MRI scanners for claustrophobic or very large patients. Even with fine tuning of the settings, the images from these machines are generally of lower resolution than their closed counterparts and can often make this imaging unsuitable for surgical planning purposes.

MRI has some advantages over CT imaging in that it produces direct multiplanar imaging. There is no ionizing radiation, and there is greatly increased soft tissue resolution. Figure 12.3 shows the advantage of MRI over CT imaging studies for soft tissue evaluation such as tumor definition. In addition, there is a lack of distortion from adjacent bony structures, making MRI ideal for most of the central nervous system, especially the posterior fossa and the spinal cord.

MRI has the drawback of not detailing bony structures as well as CT scan, and like CT imaging, it may be limited by artifacts caused by implants, such as metal hardware and dental implants. (Refer to Table 12.1, which outlines how to choose imaging type for some of the most common pathologies.) Until quite recently, patients with pacemakers were unable to have MRIs; however, there are now MRI-compatible pacemakers. Metal in the brain or orbits, cochlear implants, or neurostimulators are a contraindication. Body habitus, pregnancy, claustrophobia, and the inability to stay still for relatively long periods of time may make the imaging of the patient more challenging.

MRI studies can be done without or with contrast. Chelated gadolinium is used as the contrast agent in MRI studies, which is iodine free. It should still be used with caution in patients who have poor kidney function. A glomerular filtration rate (GFR) of less than 60 is considered a relative contraindication and a GFR of less than 30 an absolute contraindication for gadolinium dye. In addition, patients who are taking metformin need special consideration. Contrast-induced nephropathy can result in metformin accumulation and precipitate metformin-related lactoacidosis, a rare but recognized side effect. Patients may continue taking their metformin, but should have a creatinine level done before the imaging to ensure adequate kidney function.

■ ELECTROMYOGRAPHY AND NERVE CONDUCTION VELOCITY STUDIES

Electromyography (EMG) and nerve conduction velocity (NCV) studies are collectively referred to as EMG, although, strictly speaking, this designation should be reserved for electromyography only. Both procedures help to detect the presence and location of nerves and muscle damage due to neurological disease.

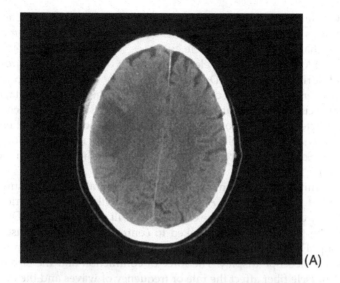

(A)

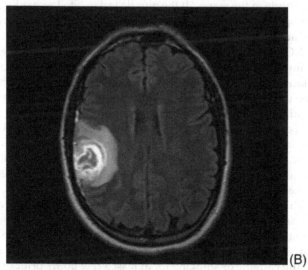

(B)

Figure 12.3 ■ Glioblastoma seen on (A) CT and (B) MRI (FLAIR sequence) imaging of the brain.

NCV detects a problem with the nerve, whereas EMG can detect diseases stemming from problems with the muscle itself or problems that influence the muscle.

EMG measures the electrical activity of muscle during rest and during contraction. During an EMG, very fine wire electrodes are inserted into a muscle to assess changes in electrical voltage that occur when the muscle is at rest and when the muscle is being contracted. The electrodes are attached to an oscilloscope, where there is a visual display of the muscle activity in the form of a wave. Sometimes there is audio output so that the activity can be heard.

Initially, the patient will be asked to relax, allowing measurement of muscles at rest. A healthy muscle will show no electrical activity during rest, and the oscilloscope will show a flat line. During the test, the patient is asked to contract a particular muscle group. Each muscle fiber that contracts produces a waveform on the oscilloscope display. The force of contraction and the size of the muscle fiber affect the rate or frequency of waves and the size or amplitude of the waves. If the muscle is damaged or has lost innervation, it may produce electrical activity during rest, and when it contracts, it may produce abnormal wave patterns.

NCV studies measure the speed of conduction of an electrical impulse through a nerve. Two sets of sticky, flat electrodes are placed on the patient at specific locations with set distances between them, allowing the examiner to pulse timed small electrical stimulus through one set of electrodes to the second set. The speed of nerve conduction is related to the diameter and the degree of myelination of the nerve. Increased conduction times indicate nerve damage. Such damage may include demyelination of the nerve, damage to the axon, or possibly a conduction block in the nerve.

There may be some discomfort with an EMG study, and the muscles where the electrodes were inserted into the muscle may bruise or ache for a few days after the test. Patients who are preparing to take an EMG or NCV test should avoid stimulants including caffeine or smoking for at least a few hours prior to the test. The use of certain medications, in particular cholinergic and anticholinergic medications, can affect test outcomes. Patients are asked to avoid aspirin and nonsteroidal anti-inflammatory for at least a day before the EMG. EMG is generally contraindicated in patients who are on antiplatelet or anticoagulation therapy (such as warfarin or Plavix) as the needle electrodes may cause bleeding into the muscle. It may also be contraindicated in people with extensive skin infections in view of the risk of spreading infection from the skin to the muscle. Testing outcomes may also be affected in patients with a large body habitus or if there is swelling of the limb being tested.

Common Neurological Symptoms and Conditions Presented in Primary Care

II

Vertigo

Vertigo is a symptom of illusory movement, commonly spin-ning, swaying, or tilting. Some sufferers perceive themselves to be in motion whereas others perceive motion of the environment around them. Asymmetry in the vestibular system causes symp-toms of vertigo. This asymmtery may be a result of damage to the labyrinth, vestibular nerve, or central vestibular structures in the brainstem or dysfunction of these structures. The patient who presents to an office visit with dizziness, vertigo, or other neuro-otological symptoms is often a challenge. There are many reasons that a patient can be experiencing such symptoms, both medical as well as neurological. There are many possible etiologies of vertigo, with the most common causes of this condition being benign par-oxysmal positional vertigo (BPPV), acute vestibular neuronitis or labyrinthitis, anxiety disorders, Ménière's disease, and migraine. Rare but important causes include vertebrobasilar ischemia and retrocochlear tumors.

The focus of this section is on neurological causes of vertigo. The provider should be well aware of other medical conditions (e.g., cardiac) that may cause similar signs and symptoms. Medi-cal causes, such as cardiac reasons, are beyond the scope of this discussion.

In this field, more than in most others, terminology for pa-tient symptomatology (dizziness, vertigo, oscillopsia, unsteadi-ness, and light-headedness) is frequently used interchangeably. To help standardize the documentation, understanding, and in-terpretation of the patient's symptoms, international consensus definitions have recently been published. Key definitions are pre-sented in Table 13.1.

Table 13.1 ■ **DEFINITIONS FOR COMMON VESTIBULAR SYMPTOMS**

Term	Definition	Possible Etiology
Vertigo	The sense of self-motion when no self-motion is occurring or the sensation of distorted self-motion during an otherwise normal head movement (internal vertigo) OR The false sense that the visual surrounding is oscillating (external vertigo)	Benign positional vertigo
		Ménière's disease
		Bilateral vestibular failure
Dizziness	The sensation of disturbed or impaired spatial orientation without a false or distorted sense of self-motion	Orthostatic hypotension
		Panic attack
Unsteadiness	The feeling of being unstable while seated, standing, or walking without a particular preference direction	Peripheral neuropathy
		Myelopathy
		Multiple sclerosis
Presyncope	The sensation of impending loss of consciousness	Cardiac
		Psychogenic
		Epileptic
Syncope	Transient loss of consciousness due to transient global cerebral hypoperfusion characterized by rapid onset, short duration, and spontaneous complete recovery	Cardiac

Source: Data from Bisdorf et al. (2009) and the Task Force for the Diagnosis and Management of Syncope of the European Society of Cardiology (2009).

■ CLINICAL APPROACHES TO VERTIGO

Of paramount importance in assessing and diagnosing patients with vestibular-type symptoms is separating the benign from the urgent–emergent diagnoses. Practically, this grossly translates into distinguishing peripheral from central nervous system lesions. Peripheral and central vertigo can usually be distinguished clinically and this distinction guides management decisions. Cannot-miss causes of new vertigo or dizziness are presented in Table 13.2.

Traditional approaches to patients with dizziness relied heavily on the premise that the type of symptom predicted the underlying etiology. Evidence now shows that the "quality of symptoms" approach is neither valid nor reliable. Evidence exists that speaks to symptom timing and triggers as being much more reliable indicators of possible etiology. As a gross rule of thumb, acute onset neurological central nervous system lesions tend to be more emergent than peripheral ones. Abrupt onset of dizziness in acute vestibular syndrome is thought to favor a vascular cause, whereas a more gradual onset, over hours, is more consistent with vestibular neuritis. In addition, vestibular symptoms that have a clear and reproducible trigger tend to have a benign etiology. There are, however, sufficient exceptions to these rules to disallow the practitioner to become complacent.

For intermittent vertiginous symptoms, the most common triggers are changes in head or body position. Common etiologies include orthostatic hypotension and BPPV (see discussion in the next section). Both may cause an unsteadiness on rising from a chair. Only BPPV, however, will cause vertiginous symptoms when rolling over in bed or reclining. Dangerous etiologies that present in a similar fashion include internal bleeding causing orthostatic symptoms.

In patients with transient dizziness, the triggers of the dizziness represent key sources of diagnostic information (e.g., BPPV

Table 13.2 ■ CANNOT-MISS CAUSES OF NEW VERTIGO OR DIZZINESS

■ Transient ischemic attack or stroke	■ Poisoning (e.g., carbon monoxide)
■ Cerebellar lesion	■ Tumor
■ Cardiac disorder (e.g., arrhythmia, pulmonary embolus)	■ Withdrawal syndromes (e.g., alcohol)
■ Miller–Fischer syndrome	■ Central nervous system infection (e.g., brainstem encephalitis)
■ Wernicke syndrome	■ Drugs (e.g., lithium)

and orthostatic hypotension are triggered by positional changes). The Dix–Hallpike maneuver is an example of a specific provocative test used to evaluate patients with transient dizziness to elicit symptoms, such as dizziness, and signs, such as nystagmus.

BENIGN PAROXYSMAL POSITIONAL VERTIGO

BPPV (sometimes also referred to as BPV), is the most common cause of vertigo. Diagnosis of BPPV is done with the Dix–Hallpike maneuver.

The symptoms of dizziness are brought on by certain head movements, such as neck extension or head rotation. A classic presentation is the onset of vertigo with lying down in bed or when rolling over while in bed. The vertiginous symptoms begin a few seconds after the triggering head movement and resolve spontaneously after a minute if the triggering movement is stopped. It is important to remember that in BPPV, the triggering action is canal specific. For example, posterior canal BPPV is triggered with tipping the head backward, not by turning the head. In addition, there is a reduction in symptoms if the same movement is performed repeatedly, although this is seldom reported as most patients avoid repeating the triggering movement.

BPPV is thought to be caused by displacement of otoliths from the vestibule of the inner ear into the semicircular canals. Although the superior and horizontal canals may be involved, it is the posterior semicircular canals that are most commonly affected.

Repositioning maneuvers such as the Epley maneuvers (outlined later in this chapter) remain the gold standard of treatment. It may take several repetitions of the maneuver to shift the otoliths and cure the disease. Identification of the side and site of the offending otoliths is important in successful treatment of the problem.

DIX–HALLPIKE MANEUVER

The Dix–Hallpike maneuver is used to diagnose BPPV. In this example, let us assume that the affected ear is on the right. With the patient sitting on the examination table, facing forward, with eyes open, turn the patient's head 45° to the right (Figure 13.1). While standing behind the patient and supporting the patient's head with one hand, rapidly move the head from an upright to "head hanging"

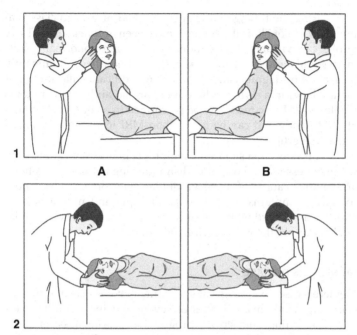

Figure 13.1 ■ (A) Dix–Hallpike positioning maneuver to the right. (B) Dix–Hallpike maneuver to the left.

where the patient's head is at least 10° below horizontal. To achieve complete dependency of the patient's head during the maneuver, the patient should be positioned in such a way that his or her shoulders will meet the head of the table when he or she is reclined.

The position is held by the patient for 30 seconds. Then the patient sits upright again and is observed for 30 seconds. The maneuver is repeated with the patient's head turned to the left (unaffected side). A positive test is indicated if any of these maneuvers cause vertigo with or without nystagmus. The side with the downward ear is the affected side in BPPV of the posterior canal.

The most common form of BPPV is caused by displacement of the otoliths in the posterior canal, causing a rotational nystagmus. An upbeating nystagmus indicates that the posterior canal is affected, and, more rarely, a downbeating nystagmus indicates that the anterior canal is affected.

Using the timing-and-triggers method of vertigo classification, four major clinical categories have been outlined (Table 13.3). Stroke can virtually be excluded if there are abnormal results in the unilateral head impulse test, direction-fixed dominantly horizontal nystagmus, and if there is no vertical ocular misalignment (skew) in a setting where there are no auditory symptoms (Table 13.4). These tests may be performed in as little as 1 minute at the bedside and can be better than MRI in ruling out central causes of vertigo.

The associated signs and symptoms that present along with the dizziness may be useful in distinguishing between peripheral and central causes of acute vestibular syndrome. General neurological symptoms or signs (e.g., diplopia and numbness) are strongly associated with central causes, but their absence is a relatively poor predictor of a peripheral cause.

MÉNIÈRE'S DISEASE

Ménière's disease is a clinical syndrome that consists of four concomitant symptoms: episodes of severe and incapacitating vertigo, fluctuating and slowly progressive hearing loss, episodic tinnitus, and aural fullness. The vertigo is usually a sensation of spinning, but can also be a feeling of being pushed or pulled, lasting on the order of several minutes to a few hours. There is a decrease in hearing that is associated with a vertigo attack, which may improve after resolution of the acute symptoms. Aural fullness refers to a sensation of plugging or clogging in the ear that also worsens when a vertigo attack begins. Many patients with ear problems will have one or all of these symptoms at some point. Patients with Ménière's disease, however, will have these symptoms occur together in discrete episodes. Between episodes, Ménière's patients feel well. This differs from many other types of vertigo and balance disorders in which the symptoms are more vague and the episodes less distinct.

The etiology of Ménière's disease is unknown, though the symptoms are thought to be produced by an increase in the fluid pressure in the inner ear. Therefore, the mainstay of treatment is directed toward decreasing the fluid pressure in the inner ear. This is done by aggressive salt restriction, sometimes in combination with a diuretic. Other treatment options are directed toward controlling the symptomatology of the disease.

Table 13.3 ■ FOUR CATEGORIES OF VERTIGO, THEIR BASIC CHARACTERISTICS, AND COMMON ETIOLOGIES

Symptom Grouping	Etiologies	Etiologic Location	Presentation
Acute, spontaneous, and prolonged (days to weeks) vestibular symptoms	Vestibular neuritis	Peripheral vestibular system disturbance	Little is known about characteristics of onset in neuritis, but some experts suggest that gradual onset over hours is typical. Sustained presentation associated with nausea and vomiting. Preserved auditory function.
	Viral labyrinthitis	Peripheral vestibular system disturbance	Similar presentation to vestibular neuritis, but distinguished by loss of auditory function.
	Posterior fossa stroke	Central nervous system lesion	Onset of dizziness is abrupt (seconds to minutes) in a large proportion of patients with stroke. Vertebrobasilar ischemic stroke may closely mimic peripheral vestibular disorders, with obvious focal neurological signs absent in more than half of people presenting with acute vestibular syndrome due to stroke.
Chronic episodic positional vestibular symptoms	Benign paroxysmal positional vertigo (BPPV)	Peripheral vestibular system disturbance	Symptoms generally last for <1 hr and are most prominent with positional changes such as rolling over in bed.

(continued)

Table 13.3 ■ FOUR CATEGORIES OF VERTIGO, THEIR BASIC CHARACTERISTICS, AND COMMON ETIOLOGIES (continued)

Symptom Grouping	Etiologies	Etiologic Location	Presentation
Chronic episodic spontaneous vestibular symptoms	Vestibular migraine	Central nervous system origin	Acute onset which may last >1 hr
	Ménière's disease	Peripheral vestibular system disturbance	
	Transient ischemic attack	Central nervous system origin	Acute
Chronic unsteadiness	Cerebellar degeneration	Central nervous system origin	Insidious
	Bilateral vestibular failure	Peripheral vestibular system disturbance	
	Spinal cord compression	Central nervous system origin	Acute or insidious

Table 13.4 ■ THE TRIAD REDICTING PERIPHERAL VERSUS
CENTRAL ETIOLOGIES

Test	Peripheral Etiology	Central Etiology
Unilateral head impulse test	Abnormal result of unilateral head impulse test	Normal head impulse tests bilaterally.
		A normal result of the horizontal head impulse test of vestibulo-ocular reflex function is the single best bedside predictor of peripheral versus central causes of acute vestibular syndrome.
Horizontal nystagmus on lateral gaze	Direction-fixed dominantly horizontal nystagmus	Direction-changing horizontal nystagmus on lateral gaze (i.e., right-beating nystagmus in right gaze and left-beating nystagmus in left gaze, with or without nystagmus when the patient looks straight ahead). This type of nystagmus generally reflects dysfunction of gaze-holding structures located in the brainstem and the cerebellum.
Skew deviation	Absent vertical ocular misalignment (skew)	Vertical ocular misalignment of vestibular causation ("skew deviation" or "skew") during the alternate cover test is generally central in origin.

More than half of the patients who develop Ménière's disease will have complete remission over time. If symptoms persist, there may be permanent damage to the inner ear resulting in hearing loss; therefore, patients with Ménière's disease should always be treated as aggressively as possible.

VESTIBULAR NEURONITIS AND LABYRINTHITIS

Vestibular neuronitis is an acute onset disruption of sensory input from one of the two vestibular apparatuses, causing an imbalance in vestibular neurological input to the central nervous system. Patients present with nausea, vomiting, and vertigo. Vestibular neuronitis is distinguished from labrynthitis by preserved auditory function despite the fact that vestibular neuronitis and labyrinthitis may be closely related in some cases.

Spontaneous, unidirectional, horizontal nystagmus is the most important physical finding. Patients may also tend to fall toward their affected side during the Romberg test or when trying to ambulate.

Vestibular neuritis is caused by a viral infection. This disease occurs most commonly in middle-aged patients. A full recovery generally occurs within a few weeks.

■ QUESTIONS TO ASK THE PATIENT

Are your symptoms continuous, waxing and waning, or sporadic, discrete episodes?

How long do the symptoms last per episode in minutes, hours, days, or months?

Have you noticed any triggering factors?

Was there a specific antecedent event to the episode of vertigo?

Was the onset of symptoms acute or insidious?

What makes the symptoms better?

What makes your symptoms worse?

Have your symptoms become worse with time?

■ USEFUL LABORATORY TESTS

No specific laboratory tests are indicated in the evaluation of vertigo. However, laboratory studies may be useful to help distinguish between vertigo and other types of dizziness such as light-headedness. For this, suggested labs would include a basic metabolic panel serum glucose, in addition to testing for anemia.

■ SPECIAL TESTING

When patients feel lightheaded, it is important to rule out cardiac involvement. Complete audiometric testing, when hearing loss is suspected, can help distinguish vestibular pathology from a retrocochlear cause, such as a schwannoma or acoustic neuroma.

Specific provocative tests such as the Dix–Hallpike maneuver are foundational in the evaluation of patients with transient dizziness to elicit symptoms (e.g., dizziness) and signs (e.g., nystagmus). However, the Dix-Hallpike maneuver and its related variants are generally unhelpful for diagnosis in patients with acute vestibular syndrome because they fail to differentiate between central and peripheral causes.

■ USEFUL IMAGING STUDIES

MRI, in particular the diffusion-weighted MRI series in acute vestibular syndrome, is useful in assessing acute lesions in the posterior fossa, a region where CT performs particularly poorly because of bone-related artifacts. It should be recognized that MRI misses up to 20% of posterior fossa strokes in the first 24 to 48 hours; despite this, it is the imaging modality of choice.

Magnetic resonance angiogram (MRA) of the head and neck is useful if a vascular cause for the symptoms is suspected.

■ TREATMENT

Most vertigo patients can be treated in the primary care setting with little diagnostic testing required. Often treatment is largely supportive as the vertiginous symptoms will resolve spontaneously with time.

REPOSITIONING PROCEDURES

Canalith repositioning procedures, such as the Epley maneuver and its variants, consist of several simple maneuvers involving positioning the patient's head. The aim is to dislodge the otoliths from the semicircular canals. Each head position is held for about 30 seconds after the vertiginous symptoms or abnormal eye movements stop. The patient must avoid lying flat or placing the affected ear below shoulder level for a week. This will mean propping the head up with some pillows while sleeping so that it is higher than the rest of the body. Patients can be taught how to do the procedure themselves so that they can do it at home.

THE EPLEY MANEUVER

This maneuver is most easily executed with the help of an assistant as it requires the patient to assume several positions while the patient's head is maintained in a fixed position. Have the assistant stand on the unaffected side of the patient. (In our example this would be on the patient's left hand side.)

With the patient sitting on the examination table, facing forward, with eyes open, turn the patient's head 45° toward the affected ear, which in our example is toward the right (Figure 13.2A).

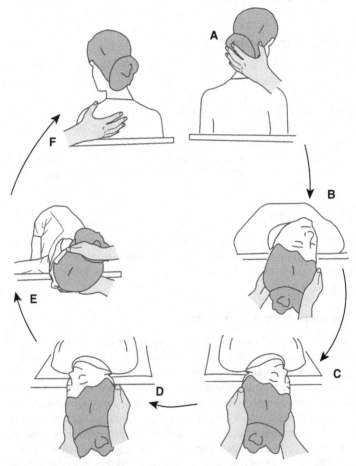

Figure 13.2 ■ The Epley maneuver.

While standing behind the patient and supporting the patient's head with one hand, rapidly move the head from an upright to "head hanging" where the patient's head is at least 10° below horizontal (Figure 13.2B). To achieve complete dependency of the patient's head during the maneuver, the patient should be positioned in such a way that his or her shoulders will meet the head of the table when he or she is reclined (this is identical to the Dix–Hallpike test).

The position should be maintained for 30 seconds or until any nystagmus and vertiginous symptoms subside (Figure 13.2C). Reposition your hands on either side of the patient's head to allow you to turn the patient's head 90° away from the affected ear, placing it at 45° toward the opposite shoulder, which in our example toward the left (Figure 13.2D). Allow any vertigo to subside before continuing.

Ask the patient to roll onto his or her shoulder on the unaffected (left) side, with the help of your assistant (Figure 13.2E). This is done by having the assistant grasp the patient's far hand and help logroll the patient toward your assistant. While the patient rolls onto his or her shoulder, maintain the patient's head at its 45° orientation to the shoulder. As the patient is rolled toward the assistant, the patient's face will be directed to the floor. Once again keep this position until the nystagmus and vertigo subside or 30 seconds have passed.

Still keeping the head turned to the left shoulder, ask the patient to sit up by first moving his or her legs off the side of the table and then raising his or her torso (Figure 13.2F). This is done with you behind the patient, maintaining the patient's head position and the assistant helping pull the patient to the seated position.

After approximately 30 seconds, the patient can resume free movement.

If necessary, the Epley maneuver may be repeated several times at 30-minute intervals if significant nystagmus or vertigo is still elicited during the Dix–Hallpike test.

There are many variations on this test.

If the canalith repositioning procedure does not work, there is the option of surgery. A bone plug is used to block the portion of the inner ear that causes the dizziness.

MEDICATIONS

Medications have limited benefit in patients with benign paroxysmal positional vertigo, because the vertiginous episodes usually last less than one minute. Medications are most useful for treating acute vertigo that lasts a few hours to several days. Vertigo lasting more than a few days is suggestive of permanent vestibular injury (e.g., stroke), and medications should be stopped to allow the brain to adapt to new vestibular input.

H1-receptor antagonists: Motion sickness medications and antiemetics may reduce the spinning sensation of vertigo and help control nausea and vomiting. The mechanism of action is thought to be in the central nervous system, possibly through central anticholinergic activity, although their exact mechanism remains unknown. Examples of such medications include dimenhydrinate (Dramamine, Dimetabs, Dymenate), diphenhydramine (Benadryl, Bydramine, Hyrexin), meclizine (Antivert), and promethazine (Phenergan).

Benzodiazepines: These medications centrally inhibit vestibular responses. Valium and ativan are most commonly used.

Anticholinergics: These work centrally by suppressing conduction in vestibular cerebellar pathways. Scopolamine is most commonly used.

Corticosteroids: Corticosteroids have many and varied activities in the body. Their anti-inflammatory properties are useful in the treatment of vertigo that is related to infection or inflammation. They reduce inflammation of the vestibular nerve and its associated apparatus, leading to faster recovery and less permanent damage. Steroid treatment should be used judiciously, given the large side-effect profile.

Diuretics: For the treatment of Ménière's disease, diuretic medication reduces fluid retention, thereby lowering pressure in the inner ear. This results in fewer episodes and less severe symptoms of Ménière's disease. Patients on long-term diuretics may need potassium supplementation.

PHYSICAL THERAPY

A physical therapist trained in vestibular disorders can teach a patient useful techniques to improve his or her symptoms and functionality. For example, with BPPV the patient can learn canalith repositioning techniques to do at home. A patient may be taught to avoid vertigo-triggering movements, for example, avoiding lowering his or her head when bending down to pick something up from the floor and bending his or her legs instead. There are also various exercises that help improve balance.

HOME REMEDIES

Patients with BPPV may be counseled to sleep with their head slightly higher than the rest of their body. This can be done by simply propping up their head and shoulders with some extra pillows. It is prudent to discuss with the patient the avoidance of known patient-specific triggers as well as general triggers that may make symptoms worse, such as bright lights, reading, sudden movements, or watching TV. A patient should be strongly counseled to stop smoking. Patients who quit smoking experience fewer episodes of vertigo with less severe symptoms.

Tremor

A tremor is a type of involuntary shaking movement with an associated rhythm. A tremor is most often noticed in the hands, but it may affect any body part, including the head, voice, body, or lower extremities. The pathophysiology of tremors is poorly understood. Broadly speaking, tremors may derive from four sources:

1. Mechanical oscillations of the limb, which occur at a particular joint. The tremor arises through the natural mechanical tendency for body parts to oscillate at certain frequencies.
2. Mechanical reflex oscillations, which are a result of the inherent instability of negative muscle feedback loops in the sensory muscle pathways.
3. Normal central oscillators, which result from the fact that neural activity in the brain—in particular the thalamus, basal ganglia, and inferior olive—is strongly rhythmic in nature.
4. And finally, pathologic central oscillations, which arise from the same structures in the central nervous system as the normal central oscillations, namely the thalamus, basal ganglia, inferior olive, and cerebellum.

It is likely that various combinations of these mechanisms are simultaneously involved in producing tremor in both the healthy and the ill patient.

The speed of the tremor is referred to as its frequency and is measured in Hertz (Hz). A low-frequency tremor is in the range of 3 to 5 Hz, a medium-frequency tremor is in the range of 6 to 12 Hz, and a high-frequency tremor is more in the range of 12 to 18 Hz. The size of the tremor is known as its amplitude. Amplitude may be broadly spoken of as coarse (large amplitude) or fine (small amplitude).

■ CLINICAL APPROACH TO TREMORS

Observe the patient to determine whether the tremor occurs primarily with action or at rest. A very fine tremor may be evaluated by asking the patient to hold his or her arms straight out in front with palms down, and then placing a piece of paper on the outstretched hands, making the tremor easier to see. Check for symmetry of the tremor and for associated symptoms such as weakness, sensory changes, and reduced or heightened reflexes. A detailed history should be taken, including family history of tremors, and changes in handwriting, dexterity, or grip strength should also be investigated.

Tremors can be divided on an etiologic basis or according to clinical findings. Clinical findings are classified by whether the tremor occurs at rest or with movement/posture, tremor frequency, and tremor amplitude. Some of the most common forms of tremor are described here and summarized in Table 14.1

PHYSIOLOGIC TREMOR

Physiologic tremor is a medium (10 Hz) frequency fine tremor that is barely visible to the naked eye. It is present in every normal person while maintaining a posture or movement. The movement is so fine that it is only perceptible when arms are outstretched and fingers held taut. Neurological examination results of patients with physiologic tremor are usually normal. A physiologic tremor may be present during waking hours as well as sleep. Pathologic tremors are present only during waking hours.

ENHANCED PHYSIOLOGIC TREMOR

Enhanced physiologic tremor is a medium-frequency, coarse tremor that occurs primarily when a specific posture is maintained. It is pathologic in its amplitude and can interfere significantly with a patient's activities of daily living. Anxiety, metabolic disturbances, withdrawal syndromes, drugs, and toxins may also cause this form of tremor. Enhanced physiologic tremor can improve when the underlying etiology is resolved.

Table 14.1 ■ COMMON TREMORS AND THEIR BASIC CHARACTERISTICS

Tremor	Most Noticeable With	Distinctive	Frequency	Comments
Physiologic tremor (postural)	Isometric muscle contraction	Bilateral, barely perceptible to the naked eye with outstretched hands	Medium (10 Hz)	Benign condition thought to be a fusion of peripheral and central rhythmic cycling.
Postural and action tremor	Isometric muscle contraction	Present in active movement and absent when limbs are at rest	Medium (10 Hz)	Present when limbs and trunk actively maintain certain positions, especially as greater precision of movement is demanded.
Enhanced physiologic tremor	Isometric muscle contraction	Physiologic with exaggerated amplitude of tremor	Medium (8 Hz)	Also known as a physiologic tremor of pathologic amplitude.
Essential tremor	Deliberate action	Bilateral	Low to medium (4–8 Hz)	There may be a family history of tremor.
				Alcohol intake may reduce the tremor. Progressive in nature. Both peripheral and CNS involvement.

(continued)

Table 14.1 ■ COMMON TREMORS AND THEIR BASIC CHARACTERISTICS (*continued*)

Tremor	Most Noticeable With	Distinctive	Frequency	Comments
Parkinsonian	At rest	May be unilateral	Low (3–5 Hz)	Classically seen as a "pill-rolling" action of the hands that may also affect the chin, lips, legs, and body, can be markedly increased by stress or emotions. Tremor may initially be unilateral and then progress to the other side of the body.
Intention (ataxic or cerebellar)	Most focused portion of an action	Irregular in more than one plane	Low (3–4 Hz)	A kinetic tremor that is present when the most demanding portion of a movement is made.
				This tremor is associated with cerebellar disease.
Holmes (ataxic rubral)	Any movement	Irregular, may be large action	Low (3–6 Hz)	Due to midbrain lesions in the vicinity of the red nucleus. There may be a delay between the lesion and onset of the tremor.
				Signs of ataxia and weakness may be present. Common causes include cerebrovascular accident and multiple sclerosis.

Drug-induced	Combination of kinetic, postural, and resting	Bilateral	Medium (10 Hz)	Tremor depends on the patient and the drug used. May resolve with withdrawal of the offending agent.
Systemic illness	Deliberate action	Bilateral	Medium (10 Hz)	Tremor may present along with other disease symptoms. May resolve with resolution of illness.
Orthostatic	On standing	Bilateral lower extremities	High (>12 Hz)	This type of tremor occurs in the legs immediately on standing and is relieved by sitting down. There are typically no other clinical signs or symptoms present.
Psychogenic	Combination of kinetic, postural, and resting	Varied	Varied	Psychogenic tremor decreases with distraction. Unlike other tremors, psychogenic tremor does not diminish with loading of the affected limb. This is a diagnosis of exclusion.

ESSENTIAL TREMOR

Essential tremor is a low-frequency physiologic tremor. There are many subtypes of essential tremor. Classic essential tremor is predominantly kinetic, seen when the patient engages the muscles to execute a deliberate action. Familial essential tremor is inherited in an autosomal dominant pattern with near 100% penetrance and cannot be distinguished clinically from other forms of essential tremor. Both men and women are equally affected by familial essential tremor. This tremor becomes evident later in life and is progressive in nature, becoming quite debilitating in certain patients.

PARKINSONIAN TREMOR

The parkinsonian tremor is coarse and rhythmic in nature with a low frequency, frequently referred to as a pill-rolling-type tremor. It is characterized by being present at rest, and virtually dissipating with action. It typically affects the hands, although it may also affect the chin, lips, legs, and body, and can be greatly increased by stress or emotions. The tremor may affect the patient in an asymmetric fashion. Frequently, a Parkinsonian tremor will start in one limb or on one side of the body and progress to the other side.

INTENTION TREMOR

Intention tremor, also known as an ataxic or cerebellar tremor, is seen with deliberate and precise movement. The tremor is absent during the initial part of the action and becomes apparent during the most intense portion of the action, such as touching the tip of the nose or raising a spoon to the mouth. Holmes' tremor, also known as a rubral tremor, is a most debilitating form of intention tremor owing to the exaggerated amplitude of the tremor, that can be large enough to throw a person off balance.

DRUG-INDUCED AND SYSTEMIC ILLNESS TREMOR

The signs and symptoms of drug-induced tremors depend on the patient and the drug used. This tremor may resolve with withdrawal of the offending agent.

Tremors due to systemic illness often have associated symptoms, which include asterixis, mental status changes, and other signs of systemic disease. Thyrotoxicosis and hepatic failure are among the common causes. These tremors generally resolve with resolution of the illness.

ORTHOSTATIC TREMOR

Orthostatic tremor occurs in the legs with standing and is relieved by walking or sitting down. There are typically no other clinical signs or symptoms present. An orthostatic tremor is a high-frequency tremor that is more easily felt than seen.

PSYCHOGENIC TREMOR

Psychogenic tremors are the most varied in presentation and can therefore be a challenge to diagnose. Typically, they are acute in onset and can involve any part of the body, but they most commonly affect the extremities. Psychogenic tremor decreases with distraction and is associated with multiple other psychosomatic complaints. A psychogenic etiology for tremor is determined by a process of systematic exclusion.

Not all tremors correspond exactly with those described here, and there may be variations in the presenting symptoms. Tremors are also not mutually exclusive, and multiple tremor types may present simultaneously—for example, a patient with essential tremor may also develop a drug-induced tremor from lithium or a parkinsonian tremor.

■ QUESTIONS TO ASK THE PATIENT

Where is your tremor (hand, voice, head, legs)?

Does the tremor improve or become worse with movement?

When did you first notice the tremor?

Has your tremor become worse over time?

Have you noticed any associated symptoms?

Is the tremor continuous or intermittent?

Is there a pattern associated with the tremor (time of day, fatigue, medications)?

Are there any associated symptoms (nausea and vomiting, confusion, gait changes, anxiety, or panic attacks)?

What makes the tremor better (rest, alcohol)?

What makes the tremor worse (reaching for objects, sitting still, maintaining a specific position)?

Is there a family history of tremor?

■ USEFUL LABORATORY TESTS

The suspected etiology of the tremor will guide whether (and what) tests may prove to be useful in diagnosis and treatment. In most cases, a basic metabolic panel (BMP), complete blood count with differential (CBC/diff), and thyroid function tests set a baseline for workup. In cases of suspected drug or alcohol intoxication, specific panels may be ordered. For example, lithium is known to have a narrow therapeutic index, and when a person is taking lithium, it should always be considered as a potential offending agent. The same is true for many of the anticonvulsants, as well as recreational drugs and alcohol, although with chronic alcohol use the patient may have a tremor without an elevated alcohol level, or when the patient stops drinking.

Systemic illness may call for basic labs as indicated previously and then additional lab tests in the form of C-reactive protein and erythrocyte sedimentation rate (ESR), which are markers of inflammation. An elevated white blood cell count is a red flag; be aware, however, that certain drugs (such as lithium) may cause leukocytosis in the absence of infection.

There are no specific tests for many of the other tremor states, including Parkinson's disease. In this case, laboratory studies may be useful in excluding certain diagnoses, thereby narrowing the differential.

■ USEFUL IMAGING STUDIES

No specific imaging studies are recommended for the diagnosis of tremor. MRI studies may prove useful as part of a stroke workup if stroke is a suspected cause of tremor, but not for the sake of tremor itself.

■ **TREATMENT**

There are four main treatment paths that may be considered in the treatment of tremor:

1. **Removing any offending agents**, such as drugs, alcohol, or other toxic compounds, or treating any systemic illness. Many times if the etiology can be resolved, such as removing offending drugs, the tremor will spontaneously resolve. In such cases, that is the treatment of choice.
2. **Lifestyle interventions**, such as limiting caffeine intake or other stimulants, meditation to reduce stress, biofeedback, psychotherapeutic counseling for psychogenic tremor, and physical therapy to improve coordination and control. Alcohol has some benefit in reducing essential tremor, but this treatment modality needs to be balanced by the risks of regular alcohol intake.
3. **Drug treatment** of tremors, including dopamine-like drugs, beta blockers, amantadine, anticholinergics, benzodiazepines, anticonvulsants, and botulinum toxin. Precise diagnosis of the tremor is paramount in selecting the pharmacologic agent.
4. **Surgical intervention**, such as deep brain stimulation or thalamotomy, may ease certain tremors. When a tremor is severe and no longer responds adequately to medical management, surgical options can be explored. Response can be excellent.

Low Back Pain 15

Low back pain is a common problem but, in most cases, one with no good treatment. Care must be taken to differentiate the (important) minority of patients with significant pathology and potentially catastrophic disorders, such as epidural spinal cord compression, from the vast majority of patients who can be successfully managed at home. The majority of back pain is caused by musculoskeletal/ligamentous strain or osteoarthritis. These causes are not emergent and may be managed with home remedies, such as heat and ice, nonsteroidal anti-inflammatory treatment (NSAIDs), and physical therapy. These patients are expected to return to normal activity within a relatively short period of time.

When evaluating a patient with back pain with or without radicular symptoms, pay attention to whether the symptoms are indicative of systemic disease or whether they are more focal, indicating a localized musculoskeletal or mechanical problem. In treating back pain, it is also important to assess the patient for signs of psychosocial issues that may augment symptoms and prolong the natural course of the disease. This can be a confounding factor in assessment and diagnosis of the patient with back pain.

■ CLINICAL APPROACH TO LOW BACK PAIN

The assessment of a patient with low back pain starts by examining the gait of the patient as he or she walks into the clinic or examination room (please refer to Chapter 10 for further discussion of gait and gait changes). Inspect the patient's back for scoliosis, asymmetry, coronal and sagittal balance, and unusual hair growth, especially a tufting at or just above the gluteal cleft. The spine may be palpated for muscle tone, spasm, or atrophy as well as localized bone pain or warmth. Finally, assess the patient by examining the patient's gait (if this was not done before) and ability to heel, toe, and tandem walk. Have the patient touch his or her toes, hyperextend, and lateral bend to test for range of motion. Be sure to determine whether the patient is guarding for pain or whether he or she has a true reduction in the range of motion. Assess strength, sensation, and reflexes (please refer to Chapters 7 to 9 for more detailed information). Finally, have the patient lie supine to allow for testing of a straight leg raise test and other provocative tests as described later in this chapter.

MUSCLE STRAIN AND SPRAIN

The lumbar spine bears much of the body's weight; strains and sprains of the lower back, therefore, are common. Twisting or pulling a muscle or tendon causes back strain, whereas pulling and tearing ligaments causes a back sprain.

Typically, muscle strain and sprain will present as pain that intensifies with movement, muscle cramping or spasms (sudden uncontrollable muscle contractions), and decreased function or range of motion of the joint. Muscle sprain and strain may result in difficulty walking, bending forward or sideways, or standing straight.

Lumbar strains and sprains may be caused by repetitive actions or a single instance of improper lifting, both of which cause overstressing the back muscles. This is especially true if the patient is undertaking an activity that is not part of his or her normal daily routine. Chronic lumbar strains usually result from repetitive movement of the muscles and tendons over longer periods of time.

Patients are more at risk for lumbar strains and sprains if they have excessive lordosis (curvature) of the lumbar spine, are overweight, have poor core strength, or have tight hamstring muscles. Sports that can place a patient at risk for these injuries include those that involve twisting or pulling, such as weightlifting.

Mild to moderate strains and sprains may be diagnosed on the patient's history of present illness and physical exam. More severe strains and sprains may warrant some imaging such as plain films to rule out fracture or listhesis.

TROCHANTERIC BURSITIS

Trochanteric bursitis is inflammation of the trochanteric bursa (Figure 15.1) on the lateral aspect of the upper thigh over the greater trochanter. Typically, trochanteric bursitis presents as pain on the outside of the hip and thigh or in the buttock, especially noticeable with palpation. The pain from trochanteric bursitis increases with activities that put pressure on the bursa, such as getting up from a deep chair, or getting out of a car, or pain with walking up stairs. Lying on the affected side also increases the pain. Trochanteric bursitis may be a result of direct injury to the greater trochanter, overuse or injury to the hip, incorrect posture, or postural compensation for a comorbidity causing stress of the soft tissues due to poor joint positioning, although in rare cases infection may also be a cause, or it may be idiopathic.

Bursitis is most common in women and middle-aged or elderly people. Trochanteric bursitis can remain incorrectly diagnosed for years because it shares the same pain pattern with many other musculoskeletal conditions.

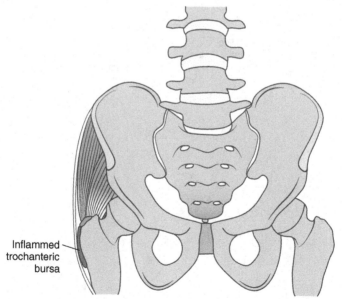

Inflammed trochanteric bursa

Figure 15.1 ■ Trochanteric bursitis (inflammation of the trochanteric bursa).

Bursitis is best treated with resting the affected area by modification of activities to reduce the overuse of that area. Physical
therapy is the mainstay of treatment to help strengthen and stabilize the associated joints and should include hamstring stretching, core strengthening, postural training, and posterior column
strengthening. The use of NSAIDs is helpful, and cortisone shots
into the bursa may be considered for more severe cases. Surgical
resection of the trochanteric bursa yields mixed results with no
supporting evidence-based data.

SACROILIITIS

The sacroiliac joints (SI joints) lie between the sacrum and the ilium,
connecting the spine to the pelvis and lower skeleton (Figure 15.2).
When compared with other joints such as the hip or the knee, these
joints have minimal movement. The sacroiliac joints are stabilized
with ligaments that when damaged can lead to too much motion
in the joint, resulting in inflammation of this joint, which is known
as sacroiliitis.

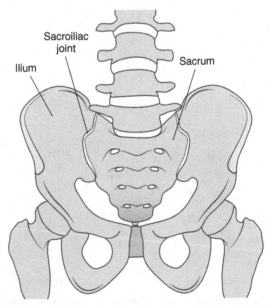

Figure 15.2 ■ Sacroiliitis (inflammation of the sacroiliac joint).

Leading causes of sacroiliitis include degenerative arthritis; traumatic injury to the buttock or pelvic region; pregnancy and childbirth, as a result of the pelvis widening and stretching the SI joints during childbirth; or infection of the SI joint or other systemic infections. Inflammatory conditions of the spinal column may also cause SI-joint inflammation. As a group, these conditions and diseases are termed spondyloarthropathy and include conditions such as ankylosing spondylitis, psoriatic arthritis, and reactive arthritis. Sacroiliitis may also be a component of other types of rheumatological conditions such as ulcerative colitis, Crohn's disease, or osteoarthritis.

Patients with sacroiliitis will complain of low back, buttock, and thigh pain. This pain, or sometimes stiffness, worsens with prolonged sitting or when getting out of bed in the morning. The Patrick, or FABERE, test specifically tests for hip and SI joint pathology, as described above. Gaenslen sign is specific for testing SI joint function, but may be difficult to execute with heavier or less mobile patients.

The cornerstone for treatment of sacroiliitis is physical therapy focused on an SI joint stabilization protocol. For severe cases, SI joint steroid injections may be considered.

FABERE TEST (PATRICK TEST)

Patrick test or FABERE test (an acronym for Flexion, ABduction, External Rotation, and Extension) is performed to evaluate pathology of the hip joint and the SI joint.

Have the patient lie supine and relaxed, allowing you to place the heel of his or her foot on the knee of the opposite leg (Figure 15.3). The hip joint is now flexed, abducted, and externally rotated. Inguinal pain elicited on the ipsilateral side as the flexed hip is a sign of hip or surrounding muscle disorder. In this position, the SI joint may now be stressed by placing pressure on the flexed knee while simultaneously pressing on the anterior superior iliac spine on the opposite side. Pain in the buttocks or the lumbosacral area with this movement is indicative of SI joint pathology.

As back pain, SI joint pain, and hip pain may have very similar presenting symptoms, the examination of the lower back should be performed in concert with examination of these other areas to rule out referred symptomology.

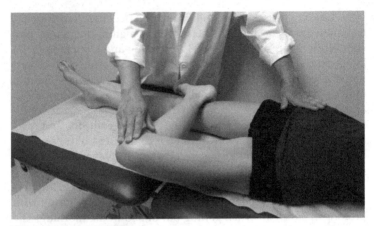

Figure 15.3 ■ FABERE test.

GAENSLEN SIGN

The patient lies supine on the examination table and is asked to draw his or her legs up to the chest. The patient is then shifted to the edge of the examination table, such that one buttock extends over the side of the examination table. The corresponding foot is then dropped unsupported, allowing it to dangle off the edge of the examination table (Figure 15.4). Pain with this maneuver is indicative of SI joint dysfunction.

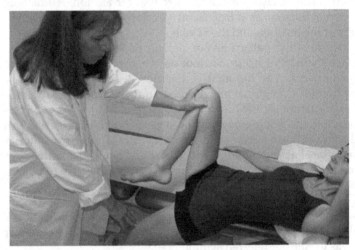

Figure 15.4 ■ Gaenslen's sign.

PIRIFORMIS SYNDROME

Piriformis syndrome is a peripheral neuritis of the sciatic nerve usually associated with spasm of the piriformis muscle and compression or irritation of the sciatic nerve (Figure 15.5). This results in pain and/or paresthesias along the tract of the sciatic nerve from the buttocks and into the leg. This syndrome is often overlooked in clinical settings because its presentation may mimic other syndromes, including lumbar radiculopathy or trochanteric bursitis.

Symptoms may be of sudden or gradual onset. The most common presenting symptoms of piriformis syndrome is increasing pain after sitting for longer than 15 to 20 minutes, walking, or sitting cross-legged. Many patients complain of pain through their buttocks, most notably over the area of the muscle's attachments at the sacrum and medial greater trochanter. Patients may also experience pain through the SI joint region, greater sciatic notch, and piriformis muscle. The pain may radiate to the knee. There is no validated test for piriformis syndrome, but it should be considered when there is sciatic-like pain without a clear spinal etiology.

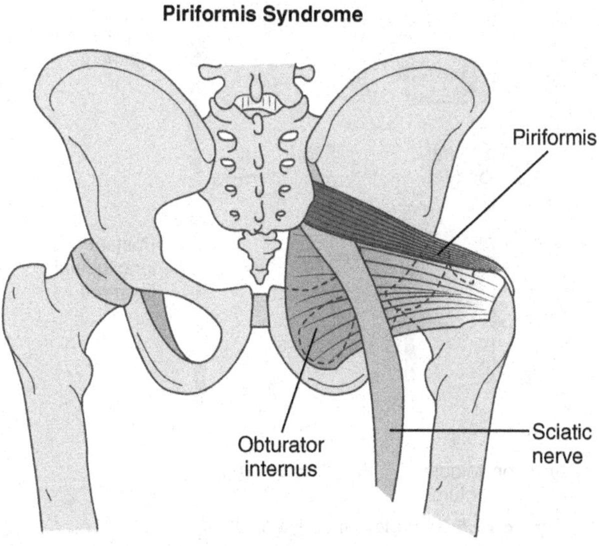

Piriformis Syndrome

Figure 15.5 ■ The piriformis muscle and sciatic nerve.

COMPRESSION FRACTURES

Compression fractures have three etiologies: trauma, fractures of insufficiency (osteoporosis), or fractures from metastatic disease. Fractures of insufficiency are a result of osteoporosis, which may stem from underlying issues such as renal or liver disease or prolonged use of corticosteroids. Compression fractures may be classified according to where the damage occurs on the vertebral body and the extent of damage. When referring to the location of damage, the vertebral body can be divided into three "columns": anterior, middle, and posterior (Figure 15.6). Simple compression fractures involve only the anterior elements of the vertebral body, whereas more complex fractures may involve the middle and posterior elements as well.

Pain is the overriding complaint for patients who have experienced a vertebral fracture, and it can be blinding, especially

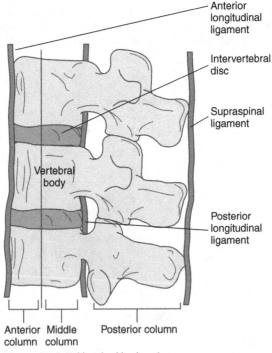

Figure 15.6 ■ Vertebral body columns.

when the patient moves to change position, such as rolling over in bed, or getting up out of bed or a chair. Hyperextension helps relieve the pain as it places more of the body weight on the posterior spinal elements and away from the anterior aspect of the spinal column. Pain can be expected to resolve between 6 weeks and 3 months, although some people do not experience pain or have symptoms for only a few weeks postinjury. Intractable pain may be a reason for surgical intervention.

OSTEOPOROTIC COMPRESSION FRACTURES

Osteoporotic compression fractures most commonly are simple compression fractures that often follow low energy trauma in elderly patients (Figure 15.7). In fact, there may be no trauma at all—simply reaching for something in the refrigerator or sitting down on a chair may be enough. Nonsurgical intervention is the first-line treatment for these fractures and includes bracing and pain control. Also, if the patient has poor bone density, the underlying cause of the osteoporosis is addressed. A hyperextension brace may provide significant pain relief, but can be difficult to fit on elderly patients who have a severe underlying kyphosis or have pulmonary insufficiency such as chronic obstructive pulmonary disease (COPD). Elderly patients who are minimally mobile may not benefit from bracing. Narcotic pain medication should be used with caution in the elderly.

Intractable pain, failure to heal with nonsurgical treatment, neurological deficits, or progression of the kyphosis at the fracture site are indications for surgical intervention. Vertebroplasty and kyphoplasty are the two minimally invasive surgical interventions for osteoporotic compression fractures without spinal canal compromise. Advanced patient age, the presence of comorbid conditions, and difficulty of hardware placement in weakened osteoporotic bone make more aggressive surgical intervention an absolute last resort.

ACUTE TRAUMATIC COMPRESSION FRACTURES

Acute traumatic compression fractures are the result of axial loading on a flexed spine. The anterior column fails, causing compression of the anterior aspect of the vertebral body, while the middle column remains intact. The posterior column may or may not fail, depending on the energy level of the injury. Posterior column

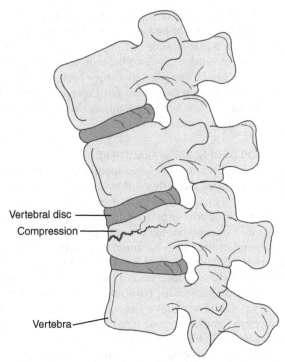

Vertebral disc —

Compression —

Vertebra—

Figure 15.7 ■ Simple compression fracture.

ligamentous integrity is the primary determinant of spinal stability in acute traumatic compression fractures. Simple compression fractures are wedge-shaped with no loss of posterior body height and no involvement of the posterior elements of the vertebral bodies.

It is important to ensure that it is a simple wedge compression fracture and not a burst fracture (as described in the following). If in doubt arrange a CT, as posterior element involvement is best determined with CT imaging.

In the absence of neurological injury or clear evidence of instability, nonoperative treatment is the preferred method of treatment. The patient's age, general health, lifestyle, and body habitus should be considered when choosing a treatment plan. Treatment involves bracing and pain control with careful follow-up to detect progressive kyphosis. Progression of the vertebral body deformity or new-onset neurological deterioration is indicative of instability and should be addressed more aggressively. CT or MRI findings of fracture progression resulting in further canal compromise, concurrent with neurological deficit, provide a strong incentive for surgical decompression and stabilization.

BURST FRACTURES

Burst fractures are more unstable than compression fractures. They involve an injury to the middle or posterior columns (or both), and may be associated with retropulsion into the spinal canal (Figure 15.8). Because there is some degree of canal compromise, there is a correspondingly greater risk of neurological injury.

The integrity of the posterior column, the extent of vertebral body collapse, and the resulting kyphosis contribute to the overall stability of the spinal column and are taken into account when deciding between surgical and nonoperative treatment. For the patient with a no neurological deficit, nonsurgical treatment may be adequate. Nonsurgical treatment involves bracing with a well-molded thoracolumbarsacral orthosis (TSO) for 3 months, pain control, and early mobilization. The argument for surgical intervention is that

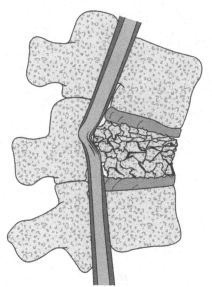

Figure 15.8 ■ Burst fracture with retropulsion into the spinal canal.

surgery will decompress the spinal canal, preventing the development of spinal stenosis. However, the spontaneous resorption of retropulsed bone has been documented in patients who have been treated nonoperatively with bracing. Complications associated with prolonged reduced mobility favor surgical intervention with the goal of early mobilization of the patient. Patients with progressive neurological deficits should undergo surgery.

PARS DEFECTS

A pars defect is a break (spondylolysis) in one of the bony bridges that connects the upper with the lower facet joints (Figures 15.9 and 12.2). A pars defect may be a result of a congenital malformation or, more commonly, of a stress fracture. The vast majority of spondylolitic defects occur at the L5 level. A pars defect can either be asymptomatic or associated with significant low back pain. Where a pars defect is associated with spondylolisthesis (slippage of one vertebral body on another) and is symptomatic, surgical intervention may be warranted.

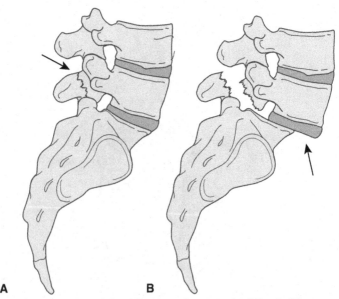

A   B

Figure 15.9 ■ Pars defect (A) with resultant spondylolisthesis (B).

There is an increased prevalence in men and athletes participating in certain high-risk sports. The most common sports that cause a problem are those with a high incidence of hyperextension and rotation such as gymnastics, weightlifting, wrestling, and dancing.

NERVE ROOT COMPRESSION

The lumbar roots emerge from below the pedicle of their respective vertebra, just above the disc. For example, the L4 nerve root exits the neural foramen just above the L4-5 disc. The descending roots are most vulnerable just above their exit foramina, as they are then the most anterior and the most lateral root in the spinal canal lying in the immediate path of a lateral disc herniation. Since the L4 root emerges above the L4-5 disc, a lateral herniation of the L4-5 disk will impinge on the descending L5 root (Figure 15.10).

Compression of a nerve root can cause significant radicular pain, which follows a dermatomal distribution. (For more on dermatomal sensory mapping, please refer to Chapter 8.) The pain may be associated with paresthesia (such as pricking or tingling; heightened sensitivity) or sensory loss in the same dermatomal distribution, and there may also be a loss of power in the muscles innervated by the nerve root (myotomal patterning). (For more on myotomes, please refer to Chapter 7, where there is in-depth guidance on testing each myotome.) This is a burning or electric-type pain that radiates down the limbs; there may be an underlying constant ache.

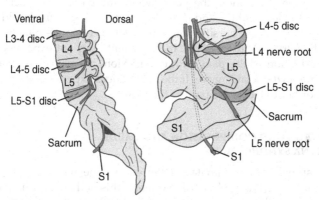

Figure 15.10 ■ L5 nerve root compression due to L4-5 disc protrusion.

Intervertebral disc protrusions are the most common source of a compressive radiculopathy, although a radiographic finding of a disc protrusion in and of itself does not signify the necessity for medical or surgical intervention. The natural history of most disc protrusions is self-limited. At least half the population of people under 60 have disc protrusions on MRI and are asymptomatic. Clinical correlation to radiographic findings is, therefore, important. Lumbar intervertebral disc herniation occurs most commonly at L4-5 (L5 root) and at L5-S1 (S1 root) interspace.

STRAIGHT LEG RAISE

A straight leg raise test is designed to reproduce back and sciatic leg pain (L5 distribution), and is used as part of the diagnostic process. Have the patient lie supine and relaxed with both legs straight. While supporting the patient's foot at the heel, have the patient allow you to passively raise first one leg and then the other (Figure 15.11A). The knee should remain straight. To ensure that it does, place your other hand on the anterior aspect of the knee as the leg is raised. If the straight leg raise causes pain, determine whether the cause is the sciatic nerve or hamstring tightness or hip pain by asking the patient to locate the place and type of pain that he or she is experiencing. A positive straight leg raise may cause back pain or pain anywhere along the sciatic nerve. Typically, this is a sharp shooting pain in a sciatic (L5-S1) distribution. The patient may also complain of pain in the opposite leg, which would be a positive crossed straight leg raise test. When slowly raising the patient's leg, note the point where the pain is experienced, lower the leg slightly, and dorsiflex the foot. The pain should be reproduced as the dorsiflexion of the foot once again stretches the sciatic nerve (Figure 15.11B). If the patient does not experience a reproduction of the pain with dorsiflexion, the pain is probably not due to the sciatic nerve. If the patient does experience pain, ask him or her to locate the path of the pain.

SPINAL CORD COMPRESSION AND CAUDA EQUINA SYNDROME

The spinal cord terminates at the end of the thoracic (T12) or beginning of the lumbar (L1) vertebra; this end is known as the conus medullaris. Nerve roots on each side descend past the conus within the thecal sac until they exit at the appropriate vertebral

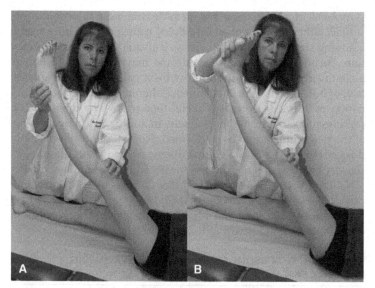

Figure 15.11 ■ Straight leg raise (A) and subsequent dorsiflexion of the foot (B).

levels. These roots are collectively known as the *cauda equina*, from the Latin "horse's tail," describing their appearance as they collectively descend. The descending nerve roots innervate the lower extremities and perineum, including bowel and bladder function.

When a mass, such as a herniated disc, is present above the conus, it causes epidural spinal cord compression and classic acute spinal cord syndrome. Such spinal cord compression frequently associated with a distinct change in sensation below the level of the lesion. Cord compression can occur at any level. Pain is the predominant presentation for patients with spinal cord compression.

When a herniated disc or other mass is present below the conus, however, the compression is on the descending nerve roots as there is no spinal cord per se to compress. The mass impinging upon the cauda equina may result in cauda equina syndrome. The hallmarks of cauda equina syndrome are "saddle" anesthesia or paresthesia (of the perineum, in a distribution similar to that which would be in contact with a saddle if one were riding on a horse), bowel incontinence, and bladder dysfunction. Cauda equina syndrome is an emergency.

Bladder dysfunction in cauda equina syndrome usually presents as difficulty initiating a urine stream or urinary retention, but in some patients may present as overflow incontinence and symptoms of a neurogenic bladder. Measurement of postvoid residuals either by placement of a Foley catheter or by ultrasound scanning should be done if there is suspicion of bladder dysfunction. Because cauda equina syndrome may present with bowel incontinence, any patient with low back pain and complaints of lack of bowel control or incontinence should have a rectal examination performed. Decreased rectal tone makes the diagnosis of cauda equina syndrome more likely. In addition, sensory testing of the perineum should be performed. Normal perineal sensation does not exclude a cauda equina diagnosis, and exam findings of sensory changes greatly increase the possibility of cauda equina.

Table 15.1 outlines some red flag findings in the history and physical examination. Any of these findings may be indicative of a more serious pathology, and advanced imaging and neurosurgical consultation should be strongly considered.

Table 15.1 ■ WORRISOME SYMPTOMS WHEN EVALUATING LOW BACK PAIN

Symptom	Concern
History of malignancy	Metastatic disease that may have spread to the spine
IV drug use	Infection as either a discitis or osteomyelitis
Recent bacteremia	Infection as either a discitis or osteomyelitis
Erythematous, focally tender, or swollen area of the lower back, suggesting a local infectious process	Cauda equina syndrome
Incontinence of bowel	Cauda equina syndrome
Perineal paresthesias	Cauda equina syndrome
Decrease in perineal sensation	Cauda equina syndrome
Decreased rectal tone	Cauda equina syndrome
Difficulty initiating a urine stream or postvoiding residual of >100 mL	Cauda equina syndrome
Bilateral leg symptoms	Cauda equina syndrome

■ QUESTIONS TO ASK THE PATIENT

Have you noticed any changes in the way that you are walking?

Have you noticed any new trouble with your balance?

Do you have a history of malignancy?

Do you have a history of intravenous drug use or recent bacteremia of any cause?

Are you incontinent of bowel?

Do you have any bladder dysfunction, whether inability to start a urine stream or incontinence?

Do you have "saddle" paresthesias or anesthesia?

Have you had fever or chills?

Are your symptoms the same on the left as on the right?

■ USEFUL LABORATORY TESTS

No specific laboratory tests are indicated in the initial evaluation of low back pain.

■ USEFUL IMAGING STUDIES

X-rays or CT scan images are useful for visualization of the bony structures of the lumbar spine. It is not necessary to do a CT scan initially unless there is concern over complex bony issues, such as a traumatic fracture of the posterior elements of the vertebral bodies or a pars defect, which would not necessarily show on a plain x-ray. A typical first step for routine workup of lumbar pain in a nontrauma outpatient setting would include plain films of the lumbar spine with anterior, posterior, lateral, flexion, and extension views. Pars defects may be more visible on oblique imaging.

MRI is warranted when soft tissue pathology is suspected, such as disc protrusions or spinal cord or nerve root impingement.

■ TREATMENT

PATIENT-CONTROLLED TREATMENT MODALITIES

Heat and ice are the lowest-cost and most easily accessible and effective treatment, which the patient can use at will and, therefore, one of the most useful first-line therapies. The patient should be cautioned not to keep either the heat or the ice in place for more than 20 to 30 minutes at a time as it can cause skin breakdown in the form of either burns or frostbite. Inflammation responds best to the use of ice, and muscle strain and fatigue respond to the use of heat. Practically speaking, the patient may simply be advised to use the modality that helps relieve their symptoms. The use of heat and ice alternately in 20 minute cycles can often break a muscle spasm and provide relief for muscle strains and sprains.

NSAIDs can be the mainstay of the treatment of low back pain both as an analgesic and as an anti-inflammatory agent. Typically, they would be taken on an "as needed" basis, but for acute episodes of low back pain, a scheduled regime of NSAIDs may be indicated. Caution should be used in the patient with gastrointestinal pathologies, in which case either switching to a cox-2 inhibitor such as Celebrex or adding a proton-pump inhibitor may be useful. Cox-2 inhibitors should not be used in patients with a cardiac history.

PROVIDER-PRESCRIBED TREATMENT MODALITIES

Oral steroids are effective agents in the treatment of low back pain where inflammation plays a role as a pain source. More than one or two courses of oral steroids in a year are discouraged owing to the side effects of steroids. In addition, consideration should be given to how often the patient takes steroids for other comorbidities.

Physical therapy (PT) centers around the right therapy for the right diagnosis. Sending a patient to PT without a clear diagnosis of the problem may be great for general conditioning and core strengthening, but may not help to relieve the patient's symptoms. For example, if a patient's final diagnosis is of a pars defect, then hamstring stretching would be imperative in the PT regime, or if the diagnosis is one of sacroiliitis, then SI-joint stabilization work needs to be done.

PT is the mainstay of treatment for many of the lumbar pathologies. It is aimed at strengthening and stabilization of the associated joints, and should include hamstring stretching, core strengthening, postural training, and posterior column strengthening.

INJECTIONS

There are a number of injections that may be given for back pain and radicular symptoms. The variations are based on location of the injection and whether the injection contains an anesthetic, a steroid, or a combination of the two.

Trigger points are focal muscles that have tightened into a knot and may irritate the surrounding nerves. A trigger point injection is aimed at relieving the tension in the muscle. If a patient can focally locate his or her back pain with one finger, trigger point injections may be appropriate. Multiple sites may be targeted. These are simple injections that can be done in the office.

Injections can focally target suspected problem areas in the spine and are done with x-ray guidance (fluoroscopy). These include interlaminar epidural steroid injections, transforaminal epidural steroid injections, selective nerve root blocks, medial branch blocks, and facet blocks. Injections can be used for both treatment and diagnostic purposes.

.

Peripheral Neuropathy

Peripheral neuropathy, a result of nerve damage to peripheral nerve cells and fibers, can affect sensory nerves, motor nerves, and autonomic nerves. Although in a peripheral neuropathy all the nerve fibers types are affected to some degree, symptoms vary, depending on which types of nerves are predominantly affected. Peripheral neuropathy may present as a mononeuropathy, involving a single nerve (e.g., carpal tunnel syndrome); polyneuropathy, involving multiple nerves simultaneously; or autonomic neuropathy, where the autonomic nerves are involved, resulting in symptoms such as abnormal blood pressure and heart rate, reduced ability to perspire, constipation, and bladder or sexual dysfunction.

Commonly, peripheral neuropathies will affect the longest nerve fibers first, starting distally and progressing proximally, leading to the well-known "glove-and-stocking distribution" descriptor of symptoms. Damage to the peripheral nervous system often leads to chronic neuropathic pain, which presents as paresthesias (pins and needles) or hyperesthesias (heightened sensation). The pain of peripheral neuropathy is generally described as tingling or burning. This pain can significantly impact a patient's quality of life and is usually difficult to treat. Occasionally, there is complete loss of sensation, which can be compared to the feeling of wearing a thin stocking or glove, or the sensation of having plastic wrap over the affected area.

The underlying causes of peripheral neuropathy include traumatic injuries, infections (such as HIV), metabolic problems, aloholism, and exposure to toxins (including certain recreational drugs). One of the most common causes is diabetes. There are many causes of peripheral nerve damage, but only three types of reactions that a nerve has to injury, namely Wallerian degeneration, axonal degeneration, and segmental demyelination.

Wallerian degeneration occurs when a nerve fiber is injured and the part of the axon distal to the injury degenerates. This reaction often occurs in focal mononeuropathies that result from trauma or nerve infarction.

Axonal degeneration, sometimes referred to as the dying-back phenomenon, results in axonal death, which starts at the most distal part of the axon. Axonal degenerative polyneuropathies are usually symmetrical, and the disease progresses in a distal-to-proximal gradient. Axonal degeneration is common in generalized polyneuropathies, such as diabetes or neuropathy from metabolic underpinnings attributed to a metabolic cause.

Segmental demyelination refers to degeneration of the myelin sheath with sparing of the axon. Demyelinating polyneuropathies are often immune-mediated or inflammatory in origin, however they can also be hereditary. Of the three types of nerve injury, segmental demyelination carries the best prognosis for recovery as remyelination restoring is accomplished more quickly than complete axonal regeneration. In peripheral nerve disorders that are characterized by either Wallerian degeneration or axonal degeneration, prognosis is less favorable because the axon must regenerate and reinnervate the underlying structure (e.g., muscle) before there is an improvement in the patient's symptoms. Recovery is more rapid with segmental demyelination because remyelination is accomplished more quickly, resulting in regeneration of the axon.

■ CLINICAL APPROACH

Peripheral neuropathy may be either inherited or acquired. Causes of acquired peripheral neuropathy include physical trauma, tumors, toxins, autoimmune responses, nutritional deficiencies, alcoholism, and vascular and metabolic disorders. Acquired peripheral neuropathies may be grouped into three broad categories. Neuropathies can be caused by (1) systemic disease, (2) trauma, and (3) autoimmune disorders and infectious disease.

Table 16.1 summarizes common neuropathies and their basic characteristics. Diabetes and hypothyroidism are common causes of chronic nerve damage. Trauma is a common cause of acute injury to a nerve. Acute trauma, such as from a motor vehicle accident, a fall, or a sports-related activity, can cause nerves to be partially or completely damaged.

DIABETES

Diabetes mellitus is a problem of elevated blood glucose, wherein the body does not produce or use insulin properly. Diabetes can lead to many acute and chronic complications. The chronic complications are mainly the result of long-standing damage to blood vessels. The major microvascular complications are diabetic retinopathy, nephropathy, and neuropathy. Diabetic neuropathy is characterized by progressive loss of nerve fibers. The exact pathophysiologic mechanism is incompletely understood, but is thought to be due to oxidative stress, increased neuronal intracellular glucose, and disruption of cellular metabolism. Diabetic neuropathy affects the large and small fiber peripheral nerves and nerves of the autonomic nervous system. Clinically, it may present in a stocking-and-glove distribution (Figure 16.1), as well as dysfunction in the autonomic neurons within the gastrointestinal tract, bladder, and blood vessels. There is no known cure for diabetes, but tight glycemic control can minimize the sequelae of this disease.

HYPOTHYROIDISM

Hypothyroidism is a disorder that occurs when the thyroid gland does not make enough thyroid hormone to meet the body's needs. Thyroid hormone regulates metabolism and affects nearly every organ in the body. Without enough thyroid hormone, many of the body's functions slow down.

Severe and chronic untreated hypothyroidism may cause a peripheral neuropathy, which is not well understood. It is thought that fluid retention that accompanies hypothyroidism may result in pressure being exerted on the nerves, resulting in nerve damage.

Table 16.1 ■ COMMON NEUROPATHIES AND THEIR BASIC CHARACTERISTICS

Neuropathy	Type	Comments
Diabetes	Systemic	Probably the most common cause of peripheral neuropathy. Progression may be slowed with tight glycemic control.
Hypothyroidism	Systemic	Not a common cause, except in severe and chronic hypothyroidism.
B₁ deficiency (thiamine)	Systemic	Thiamine deficiency, in particular, is common among people with alcoholism as they often also have poor dietary habits.
B₁₂ deficiency	Systemic	
Alcohol	Systemic	In addition to common B₁ deficiency in alcoholics, alcohol itself may cause a painful peripheral neuropathy.
Toxins	Systemic	Heavy metals (arsenic, lead, mercury, thallium), industrial drugs, or environmental toxins frequently develop neuropathy. Certain chemotherapeutic agents, anticonvulsants, antivirals, and antibiotics have side effects that can include peripheral nerve damage.
Trauma	Trauma	Acute to subacute presentation.
Lyme disease	Infectious	Wide range of neuropathic disorders, including rapidly developing, painful polyneuropathy, often within a few weeks after initial infection by a tick bite.

Herpes-family viruses: Epstein-Barr virus, cytomegalovirus, herpes simplex, and varicella-zoster (shingles)	Infectious	Virus remains latent in the nerves. Painful burning, sharp, or gnawing sensation.
HIV	Infectious	The virus can cause several different forms of neuropathy, each strongly associated with a specific stage of active immunodeficiency disease.
Acute inflammatory demyelinating neuropathy (Guillain-Barré syndrome)	Autoimmune	Acute damage to motor, sensory, and autonomic nerve fibers that may or may not reverse with time.
Chronic inflammatory demyelinating polyneuropathy (CIDP)	Autoimmune	Usually damages sensory and motor nerves, leaving autonomic nerves intact.

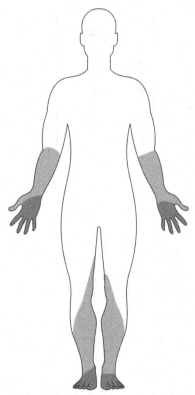

Figure 16.1 ■ Neuropathy in a glove and stocking distribution affecting the feet first and then the hands.

ALCOHOLIC NEUROPATHY AND NEUROPATHY OF POOR NUTRITION

Up to half of all long-term heavy alcohol users develop alcohol neuropathy. The cause of alcoholic neuropathy is not completely understood, but alcoholics tend to have poor nutritional status resulting in nutritional deficiencies. B_1 is essential to healthy nerve function, and B_1 deficiency is common in heavy drinkers. Vitamins E, B_6, B_{12}, and niacin are also essential to healthy nerve function. Alcohol itself may cause a painful peripheral neuropathy due to direct poisoning of the nerve. Most likely, it is a combination of direct alcohol poisoning and poor nutritional status that results in an alcoholic neuropathy.

A detailed history of alcohol and drug use should be taken from any patient presenting with a peripheral neuropathy. In addition, asking the patient about his or her nutritional status is important. Patients with alcoholic neuropathy have a longstanding history of excessive alcohol use. Symptoms are insidious in onset, chronic, and progressive. The distal lower extremities are affected first with paresthesias, dysesthesias, or occasionally weakness. Most commonly, patients will complain of paresthesias in the feet and toes first, but occasionally they will present with a history of gait ataxia or frequent falls. Interestingly, simultaneous B_1 deficiency creates a much more variable presentation of symptomology.

Physical examination findings associated with alcoholic neuropathy may include diminished sensation to vibration or pinprick stimulation in a "stocking-and-glove" distribution, as well as thermal and proprioceptive sensation abnormalities. There may be weakness on ankle or toe plantar and dorsiflexion, resulting in bilateral foot drop, with a wide-base, ataxic gait. Plantar and Achilles deep tendon reflexes are often absent or significantly reduced. The patient should be examined for additional manifestations of chronic alcohol abuse, including jaundice, gynecomastia, palmar erythema, digital clubbing, and ascites.

TOXINS

People who are exposed to heavy metals (arsenic, lead, mercury, thallium), industrial drugs, or environmental toxins frequently develop neuropathy. Certain medications, including chemotherapeutic agents, anticonvulsants, and antivirals, have peripheral neuropathy as a potential side effect.

HIV AND VENEREAL DISEASES

Neuropathy in a stocking and glove distribution is a common complication of HIV disease and can be an early manifestation of HIV infection. HIV-infected patients who use alcohol and recreational drugs are at a higher risk for developing distal symmetric polyneuropathy. Syphilis should also be considered a cause of neuropathy.

■ QUESTIONS TO ASK THE PATIENT

Describe what you are feeling in your feet/legs/arms.

Do you have pain?

Have you noticed any changes in the way that you are walking?

Have you noticed any new trouble with your balance?

Do you have a history of diabetes, alcohol abuse?

Have you been exposed to toxins or chemotherapeutic agents?

Do you have any wounds that will not heal?

Have you had fever or chills?

Are your symptoms the same on the left as on the right?

■ IMPORTANT LABS

The initial labs for determining the cause of a peripheral polyneuropathy should include a complete metabolic panel (CMP), which includes creatinine levels and liver function tests, diabetes testing, thyroid test, and testing for nutritional deficiencies. CMP testing is important as chronic alcohol consumption and illicit drug use may cause an increase in liver enzyme levels. Renal insufficiency may also be a cause of peripheral neuropathy. Peripheral neuropathy may be among the first presenting symptoms associated with diabetes mellitus (DM). Hemoglobin A1C can be used to estimate average blood glucose levels over the past 3 months. Vitamin B_1 (thiamine), vitamin B_{12}, methylmelonic acid, and folic acid levels play an important role in the proper functioning of the peripheral and central nervous systems. Nutritional deficiencies associated with alcoholism and gastric bypass surgery are common and may contribute to the development of neuropathy.

Additional laboratory tests may be ordered once more common diagnoses are excluded. These include screening for lead and other heavy metals whose toxicity is well known to cause neuropathy, testing for HIV infection and venereal disease, such as syphilis, and determining the erythrocyte sedimentation rate, which may be elevated in patients with symptoms of a peripheral polyneuropathy, owing to an inflammatory condition (e.g., paraneoplastic syndrome).

■ IMAGING

No specific imaging studies are recommended for the diagnosis of peripheral neuropathy.

■ ELECTROMYOGRAM TESTING

An electromyogram (EMG) measures the electrical activity of muscles at rest and during contraction. Nerve conduction studies measure how well and how fast the nerves can send electrical signals. Both electromyography and nerve conduction studies may be extremely helpful in the localization of nerve damage. In addition, these studies can often determine the chronicity of the nerve damage.

■ TREATMENT

MEDICATIONS

Many types of medications can be used to relieve the pain of peripheral neuropathy, including:

Over-the-counter analgesics. Mild symptoms may be relieved by over-the-counter analgesics, such as nonsteroidal anti-inflammatories (NSAIDs).

Opioids. Medications containing opioids, such as Percocet, Vicodin, oxycodone (Roxicodone), or, to a lesser extent, tramadol, can lead to dependence and addiction, so these drugs are generally prescribed only when other treatments fail.

Antiseizure medications. Medications such as gabapentin (Neurontin), topiramate (Topamax), pregabalin (Lyrica), carbamazepine (Tegretol), and phenytoin (Dilantin) were originally developed to treat epilepsy. These antiepileptics are often prescribed for nerve pain.

Capsaicin. Capsaisin is a naturally occurring substance found in hot peppers. It has been found that capsaisin has pain relieving properties causing modest improvements in peripheral neuropathy symptoms. Repeated applications are required and it may take some time and gradual exposure for the patient to get used to the burning sensation this cream causes.

Lidocaine patches. Patches that contain the topical anesthetic lidocaine (Xylocaine) may be applied to the affected area where the pain is most severe.

Antidepressants. Certain tricyclic antidepressant medications, such as amitriptyline and nortriptyline, and some serotonin–norepinephrine reuptake inhibitors (SNRIs), such as Cymbalta, Effexor, and Savella, have been found to help relieve pain by interfering with the transmission of nerve pain signals in the brain and spinal cord.

OTHER TREATMENT THERAPIES

Transcutaneous electrical nerve stimulation (TENS) is a therapy that uses adhesive electrodes, which are placed on the skin, with a gentle electric current delivered through the electrodes at varying frequencies. The patient should be encouraged to persevere with use of the TENS machine as the effect is cumulative over weeks.

People with certain peripheral neuropathy from inflammatory conditions may benefit from procedures such as plasma exchange and intravenous immune globulin, which help suppress immune system activity. Neuropathies from nerve compression, such as pressure from tumors, may need surgical resection of the tumor and nerve decompression.

New procedures are being developed such as the use of infrared therapy and magnetic therapy to help improve sensation in the feet of people with diabetes.

LIFESTYLE MODIFICATIONS

Blood glucose levels. Tight blood glucose control is important in the prevention, treatment, and control of diabetic peripheral neuropathy.

Exercise. Regular exercise may reduce neuropathic pain, improve muscle strength, improve circulation, and help control blood sugar levels. Yoga and tai chi also have been shown to help control blood sugar levels in people with diabetes and subsequently improve neuropathic pain. Massage helps improve circulation, stimulates nerves, and may temporarily relieve pain. Counsel patients not to keep their knees crossed or lean on their elbows for periods of time, because doing so may cause new nerve damage.

Nutrition. Good nutrition is especially important in patients with chronic medical conditions. A diet that is rich in fruits, vegetables, and whole grains should be encouraged.

Alcohol. Alcohol may worsen or even cause a peripheral neuropathy.

Smoking. Patients should be heavily counseled to quit smoking. Cigarette smoking can affect circulation, increasing the risk of foot problems and other neuropathic complications.

Weakness 17

Weakness is a common patient complaint, but one that is vague. The key to diagnosis starts with distinguishing the type of weakness that the patient is complaining about. Patients who present with weakness fall into three broad symptomologic categories: those with true weakness, those with weakness when challenged, and those with perceived weakness.

■ TRUE WEAKNESS VERSUS PERCEIVED WEAKNESS, FATIGUE OR EXHAUSTION

- **True weakness** (or neuromuscular weakness) describes a situation where the strength of the muscles is less than would be expected. This is the case, for example, in muscular dystrophy.
- **Induced weakness** describes conditions, such as myasthenia gravis or the metabolic myopathies, where muscle strength is normal when resting, but as the muscle is subjected to exercise it fatigues, resulting in a true weakness of that muscle. Rest allows for recovery.
- **Perceived weakness** (or nonneuromuscular) describes a situation where the patient has full strength, but feels that it requires extra effort to engage the muscle or muscle group—for example, chronic fatigue syndrome, sleep disorders, or depression.

■ CLINICAL APPROACH

When a patient initially presents with complaints of weakness, begin by asking the patient to describe his or her experience of weakness. Identifying the context and characteristics of weakness can help focus the examination process. This is important in separating out true weakness from secondary weakness or perceived weakness. In addition to primary neurological diseases that cause weakness, secondary causes of weakness include metabolic and endocrine disorders, medication effects, and psychiatric conditions. Certain features of the history of the present illness assist in narrowing the diagnosis, as outlined in the section "Questions to Ask the Patient."

Separating out fatigue from true weakness is the first step in the examination process. Diffuse feelings of fatigue are generally attributable to depression or other psychiatric conditions that prevent the patient from sustaining muscular effort. Some medications may also produce feelings of generalized weakness.

Fatigue with concurrent weakness can be caused by systemic illness such as anemic states, metabolic or endocrine disorders, vitamin deficiencies, heart disease, or cancer. Prolonged high-dose steroid use leads to reduction in muscle mass and power. This myopathy affects primarily the proximal musculature (limb and girdle muscles), leading to feelings of diffuse weakness. Severe statin toxicity occurs most commonly in a setting of polypharmacy with other medications that are hepatically metabolized.

Weakness due to cervical or upper thoracic cord compression presents in a diffuse weakness, whereas weakness as a result of nerve root compression presents in a myotomal distribution and/or with altered dermatomal sensations. Noncompressive cord lesions, such as those found in multiple sclerosis, should also be considered. Features suggesting weakness that originates in the central nervous system include altered mental status, cranial nerve involvement, and upper motor neuron signs.

There is a much higher incidence of perceived weakness in the populace than true neuromuscular weakness. Narrowing weakness into a particular myotome, being able to separate out distal from proximal weakness, as well as recognizing patterns of symptom onset and presentation can aid substantially in diagnosis. (See Chapter 7 for further discussion on myotomes.)

Weakness may arise from lesions in the central nervous system (Table 17.1). Generally, these are a result of an acute lesion and are immediately obvious to the patient with a clear etiology on evaluation. Peripheral nervous system lesions are generally more insidious and may go unnoticed (and untreated) for a considerable amount of time.

Table 17.1 ■ WEAKNESS THAT ARISES FROM LESIONS IN THE CENTRAL NERVOUS SYSTEM

Source of Weakness	Onset and Duration	Comments
CNS above the brainstem	Acute	Weakness of a limb, associated with lower facial weakness on the same side.
Brainstem lesion	Acute	Weakness of muscles on one side of the head and opposite limb. May cause complete paralysis resulting in locked-in syndrome.
Nerve root damage	Acute or chronic onset	Myotomal pattern weakness. There may be associated sensory deficits in a dermatomal distribution.
Polyneuropathy	Slow onset	Distal weakness. May be associated with sensory disturbances and changes in proprioception. Seen in diabetes, alcoholic neuropathy, and renal failure.

PRIMARY MYOPATHIES

Primary myopathies (Table 17.2) generally present as weakness of proximal muscles, namely weakness of shoulder and hip girdle muscles. They include congenital, inflammatory, and metabolic myopathies. Secondary myopathies (Table 17.2) involve those myopathies due to external sources such as infections, endocrine disturbance, drugs, toxins, and cancer. In these cases, the onset of the myopathy may be either acute or chronic.

CONGENITAL MYOPATHIES

Congenital myopathy is a term for a muscle disorder present at birth, although clinical symptoms may only appear later in an infant or child. The specific disorders are characterized on the basis of their histologic and histochemical features. These conditions are thought to be caused by genetic abnormalities of muscle development.

Congenital myopathies share common features of hypotonia, decreased deep tendon reflexes, and weakness that is greater

Table 17.2 ■ PRIMARY AND SECONDARY MYOPATHIES

Source of Weakness	Onset and Duration	Comments	Common Etiology
Primary myopathies	Chronic	Weakness of proximal muscles is suggestive of a myopathic process	Congenital or hereditary myopathies (dystrophies), inflammatory myopathies, and metabolic myopathies
Secondary myopathies Infection	Acute to chronic onset	Diffuse weakness; other symptoms are specific to etiology	Trichanosis, HIV, West Nile virus infection
Endocrine abnormality	Slow onset	Diffuse weakness	Particularly thyroid and adrenal dysfunction
Drug or toxin exposures	Acute to slow onset	Diffuse weakness	Prolonged use of high-dose corticosteroids, statin therapy especially in a setting of polypharmacy, or alcohol-induced myopathy
Cancer	Slow onset	Diffuse weakness	Most often due to cachexia, anemia, metastatic malignancy, and treatment side effects. May also be associated with depression

proximally than distally. Typically, an infant with a congenital myopathy will be flaccid with poor muscle tone, have trouble breathing or feeding, and will not progress developmentally as quickly as his or her peers.

INFLAMMATORY MYOPATHIES

The inflammatory myopathies are a spectrum of conditions that couple chronic inflammation with muscle weakness. These include polymyositis, dermatomyositis, and inclusion-body myositis. Although muscle inflammation and weakness are the universal characteristics of myopathy, there may be other associated symptoms; for instance, patients with dermatomyositis will also have a rash.

Inflammatory myopathies are acquired disorders, although there may be predisposing genetic factors. The underlying etiology in inflammatory myopathies is not clearly understood. Viruses might be a trigger for autoimmune myositis; HIV and all of the coxsackie B viruses have been implicated.

METABOLIC MYOPATHIES

Metabolic myopathies comprise a spectrum of clinically and etiologically diverse disorders caused by defects in cellular energy metabolism, which involve a diverse clinical presentation and a wide array of underlying causes. The main symptom of most of the metabolic myopathies is exercise intolerance, where the patient has difficulty with exercise and becomes tired very easily. The patient may experience fatigue, true induced weakness, painful muscle cramps, and injury-induced pain with exercising. Overexertion may cause rhabdomyolysis. The degree of exercise intolerance is very variable among patients; for some patients, formal exercise such as jogging may bring on symptoms, but for others, activities such as getting dressed in the morning or light housework may induce symptoms.

Although the metabolic myopathies characterized by exercise intolerance typically do not involve persistent muscle weakness at rest, some chronic or permanent weakness can develop in response to repeated episodes of rhabdomyolysis.

Corticosteroids may be used to preserve muscle strength in certain dystrophies, although this treatment is somewhat limited by the side effects of the medication.

MUSCULAR DYSTROPHY

The muscular dystrophies are a large group of more than 30 distinct genetic diseases characterized by progressive weakness. Muscle weakness in the dystrophies is a result of protein degeneration, which in turn leads to a degeneration of the skeletal muscles that control movement.

Among the dystrophies, there is variation in the age of onset, the sequence in which different muscle groups are affected, the extent of muscle weakness, the rate of progression, and patterns of inheritance. Muscular dystrophy occurs in both sexes and in all ages and races. The most common variety is the Duchenne variety, which most commonly occurs in young boys.

Laboratory studies may include tests for creatine kinase (CK), because where there is no trauma, high blood levels of CK suggest a muscle disease. Enzyme testing, electromyography (EMG), muscle biopsy, and genetic testing may also be indicated.

Treatments are aimed at maintaining quality of life. This is achieved by improving or preserving mobility and preventing or minimizing deterioration of deformity in joints and in the spine.

NEUROMUSCULAR JUNCTION DISEASES

Neuromuscular junction diseases are a large group of diseases that present as induced weakness, that is, a weakness that emerges when the muscle is put under stress (Table 17.3).

MYASTHENIA GRAVIS

Myasthenia gravis (MG) is a chronic, idiopathic, autoimmune neuromuscular disorder, which presents as fluctuating weakness of the voluntary muscles. MG patients have weakness that comes on with activity and improves following rest. Common symptoms include a drooping eyelid, blurred or double vision, difficulty with mouth movements resulting in dysarthria and difficulty chewing and swallowing, generalized weakness, and difficulty breathing.

It is unclear why the immune system of the person with MG makes antibodies against the nicotinic acetylcholine receptor sites of the neuromuscular junction. Acetylcholine receptor sites are involved in signal transmission for muscle movement. Decreased number of acetylcholine receptor sites due to antibody destruction causes decreased signal at the neuromuscular junction, which results in muscle weakness.

Table 17.3 ■ NEUROMUSCULAR JUNCTION DISEASES

Neuromuscular Junction Disease	Onset and Duration	Comments	Common Etiology
Myasthenia gravis	Fluctuating and episodic	Fatigue and then weakness of the specific muscles in use	Ocular symptoms are the most common presenting factor
Lambert–Eaton myasthenic syndrome	Subacute, slowly progressive	Variable fatigability of proximal muscles. Symmetric	Closely associated with systemic malignancy
Guillain–Barré syndrome	Rapidly progressive, acute and subacute presentation	Presents as an ascending weakness with loss of reflexes. Pain and paresthesias may precede the onset of weakness	Often associated with a viral infection, surgery, or trauma 1–3 weeks prior to symptom onset
Chronic inflammatory demyelinating polyneuropathy (CIDP)	Subacute, slowly progressive	Presents as an ascending weakness with loss of reflexes. Pain and paresthesias may precede the onset of weakness	A paroxysmal, chronic form of inflammatory polyradiculoneuropathy also exists

Initial testing for MG involves looking for fatigability of the involved muscle groups. Weakness with activity may be examined by having the patient do a sustained task, such as looking upward for 2 minutes, obliging the eyelids to remain elevated. In a myesthenic patient, the involved eyelid starts to droop (ptosis) (Figure 17.1). Recovery of strength after rest is then tested by allowing the patient to rest and then the same muscle group is retested to see whether strength improved with rest. For example, if one is testing for ptosis by sustained upward gaze, the patient may then rest by lying down with his or her eyes closed for several minutes with a cool washcloth over the eyelids, to determine whether eyelid function improves after rest.

MG occurs in all races, both genders, and is not age specific. It is autoimmune in nature and not thought to have any genetic or infectious component.

Laboratory testing includes antibody-specific testing. Acetylcholine receptor antibody and anti-MuSK antibody tests identify abnormal antibodies that can be measured in the blood of many people with MG.

Edrophonium (Tensilon) testing is used to differentiate MG from cholinergic crisis and Lambert–Eaton myasthenic syndrome. The administration of edrophonium prolongs the presence of acetylcholine in the synaptic cleft, resulting in significantly improved strength for the duration of the test. In cholinergic crisis, the addition of edrophonium will make the patient's weakness more profound. Lambert–Eaton myasthenic syndrome shows only marginal improvement during the Tensilon test.

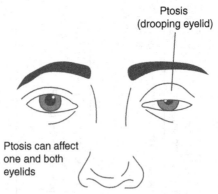

Ptosis
(drooping eyelid)

Ptosis can affect
one and both
eyelids

Figure 17.1 ■ Ptosis seen in myasthenia gravis.

EMG studies, in particular single-fiber EMG, can significantly increase the likelihood of an MG diagnosis when characteristic patterns are present.

There is no known cure for MG. First-line treatment includes medications such as anticholinesterase agents (e.g., Mestinon), which prolong the amount of time that acetylcholine remains at the neuromuscular junction. Corticosteroids, immunosuppressive agents, and intravenous immunoglobulins (IVIg) may also be used to affect the function or production of the abnormal antibodies. A patient may improve or go into remission without any specific treatment.

LAMBERT–EATON MYASTHENIC SYNDROME

Lambert–Eaton myasthenic syndrome (LEMS) is an autoimmune disease, and clinically may present in a similar fashion to MG.

Symptoms of LEMS usually begin insidiously with a slow progression. Characteristically, there is proximal muscle weakness with disproportionate involvement of the lower extremities, producing a waddling gait and difficulty elevating the arms. There may also be eyelid ptosis or diplopia, respiratory muscle weakness, depressed deep tendon reflexes, and autonomic changes. Clinically, this manifests as complaints of weakness; tender or aching muscles; difficulty rising from a chair, climbing stairs, and walking; dry mouth, eyes, or skin; constipation; or urinary retention. Anything that may cause an increase in body temperature, such as hot showers or a fever, may worsen the LEMS symptoms. LEMS has a strong association with cancer.

GUILLAIN-BARRÉ SYNDROME

Guillain-Barré syndrome (GBS) is an acute, idiopathic, inflammatory disorder of the peripheral nervous system. It is characterized by the rapid onset of weakness and, often, paralysis of the legs, arms, respiratory muscles, and face. Paresthesias and dysesthesias often accompany the weakness.

The exact cause of GBS is unknown. Some theories suggest an autoimmune trigger, resulting in damage to the myelin, leading to sensory changes and muscle weakness. More than half of GBS cases are diagnosed after an infection, surgery, or trauma, although the connection is poorly understood. Generally, it is self-limiting, but frequently the patient may be left with residual neurological deficits.

A diagnosis is often made on symptoms and clinical exam. The rapid onset of ascending weakness, frequently accompanied by abnormal sensations that affect both sides of the body similarly, is common. To confirm a diagnosis, an EMG and a lumbar puncture assessing for elevated fluid protein levels may be performed. The progression of GBS can be variable, especially early on in the acute phase, and for this reason most newly diagnosed patients are hospitalized and are admitted to the intensive care unit for close respiratory and cardiac monitoring until the disease is stabilized. The acute phase of GBS typically lasts from a few days to months. General supportive measures form the basis of care for the patient. Plasma exchange and high-dose intravenous immune globulins may be used to shorten the course of GBS. Most patients require ongoing rehabilitation after the acute phase to help regain muscle strength as nerve supply returns. GBS is indiscriminate of age, gender, or ethnic background.

CHRONIC INFLAMMATORY DEMYELINATING POLYNEUROPATHY
Chronic inflammatory demyelinating polyneuropathy (CIDP) affects the peripheral nerves and presents as a gradual and progressive weakness of the legs and, to a lesser extent, the arms. Gradual onset of symptoms, over months, as well as the chronic nature of the disease differentiate it from GBS.

Like GBS, CIDP is caused by damage to the myelin covering of the nerves, which is thought to have an underlying autoimmune etiology. Unlike GBS, however, CIDP is not self-limiting. Left untreated, one third of CIDP patients will become wheelchair bound, and so it is important to recognize and treat it early to help avoid a significant amount of disability.

Patients will present with progressive difficulty with walking worsening over several months, paresthesias or dysesthesias, and reduced or loss of lower extremity deep tendon reflexes.

Diagnosis is based on EMG studies and laboratory tests for antibodies. Treatment options are similar to those for GBS and include prednisone, high-dose IVIg, and plasmapheresis.

■ **QUESTIONS TO ASK THE PATIENT**

Describe what you mean by weak?

When did you first notice feeling weak?

Do you feel consistently weak, or do your symptoms wax and wane?

Are you weak in one area, or do you have a more generalized feeling of weakness?

Show me where you feel weak.

Does the weakness feel the same on the left- as on the right-hand side?

Do you have any other new symptoms?

Have you started taking any new medications?

Have you been exposed to any toxins or infectious agents?

■ IMPORTANT LABS

In addition to the specific laboratory tests discussed under each condition in this chapter, there are basic laboratory tests all patients should receive. These tests involved in working up most patients with symptoms of weakness initially include (but are not limited to) a complete blood count, complete metabolic panel, liver function tests, serum fasting glucose level or HbA1C, erythrocyte sedimentation rate (ESR), serum protein electrophoresis, and antinuclear antibody levels (ANA). Infectious disease tests would include HIV, Lyme titers, and venereal disease research laboratory/rapid plasma reagin tests. Nutritional tests would include vitamin B_{12} level and methylmelonic acid. In addition, toxins or heavy metal exposure testing may be indicated.

For muscle disease, creatine kinase levels in the blood are helpful because where there is no trauma, high levels of blood CK are suggestive of muscle disease. In neuromuscular disease, antibodies against acetylcholine receptors or other specific muscular antigens may be tested for.

■ EMG AND NCV STUDIES

An EMG measures the electrical activity of muscles at rest and during contraction. Nerve conduction velocity studies (NCV) measure the speed on signal conduction. Both EMG and NCV studies may be extremely helpful in the localization of nerve damage.

In addition, these studies can often determine the chronicity of the nerve damage. (See Chapter 12 on imaging and EMG studies for further discussion.)

■ BIOPSIES

For congenital myopathies, diagnosis relies heavily on muscle pathology, as laboratory testing and EMG studies may present as normal even in affected individuals.

■ TREATMENT

DIETARY CHANGES

Patients with metabolic myopathies can benefit from dietary changes. There is evidence that those with carbohydrate-processing problems may be helped by a high-protein diet, while those with difficulty processing fats may do well on a diet high in carbohydrates and low in fat.

EXERCISE

Physical therapy and exercise are important in most disease processes; this is especially true in neuromuscular disease processes. The goal is to maintain strength and slowly increase in intensity as the patient is able to tolerate it. Very weak patients who do not walk should receive range of motion exercises to prevent contractures.

For patients with metabolic myopathies who have episodes triggered by exercise or physical activity, activity may need to be modified and tailored to prevent rhabdomyolysis and the possibility of kidney damage. Each person must learn his or her activity limitations.

MEDICATIONS

Corticosteroids: Autoimmune and inflammatory-mediated neuromuscular disease may benefit from treatment with oral corticosteroid, such as high-dose prednisone. They have been shown to improve muscle strength and delay the progression of disease. These drugs have a significant side effect profile that includes osteoporosis and increased fracture risk with prolonged use. In addition, steroids can produce a steroid myopathy known as steroid myositis.

Immunosuppressants may be required in certain patients. IVIg or other immunosuppressive drugs, including cyclosporine (Neoral, Sandimmune), tacrolimus (Prograf), mycophenolate mofetil (Cellcept), and rituximab (Rituxan), may be used.

IVIg is widely used in the treatment of autoimmune neuro-muscular diseases. Compared with many of the other medication choices, such as corticosteroids or chemotherapeutic agents, it has been shown to have good therapeutic benefits with few of the side effects.

In secondary myopathies, treatment will be determined by the etiology of the disease and rectifying the underlying cause.

Dementia 18

Dementia is characterized by a significant loss of cognitive function in multiple domains that is not due to impaired arousal. The term dementia does not imply an irreversible condition, a progressive course, or a specific disease. It is an overall term that describes a constellation of symptoms associated with cognitive decline that is severe enough to interfere with daily life.

Dementia is caused by either damage to the brain or interruption of the brain's normal signaling pathways, which then produce the signs and symptoms of dementia. Different types of dementia are associated with characteristic types of brain cell damage in particular regions of the brain. Table 18.1 outlines some common causes of reversible dementias and their treatment options. Table 18.2 summarizes the most common chronic dementias.

■ CLINICAL APPROACH

There is no single test to determine whether someone has dementia. Diagnosis is based on a careful medical history, a physical examination, and laboratory tests. The medical history will elicit the characteristic changes in thinking, day-to-day function, and behavior associated with each type of dementia. The diagnosis of dementia requires either an assessment of the individual's current level of mental function and documenting a higher level of functioning in the past, or documenting a decline in mental functioning by serial examinations over a period of time (6 to 18 months). Please refer to Chapter 2 for specifics of testing a patient, available tests, and scoring of these tests over time.

Diagnosis of dementia can be made more difficult where there is focal brain disease such as a stroke, the presence of a

Table 18.1 ■ **ETIOLOGIES OF REVERSIBLE DEMENTIA**

Etiologies	Treatment
Depression	Psychiatric consult
	Psychometric testing
Medication side effects	The cost–benefit of the medication in question needs to be assessed
Excessive use of alcohol	Nutritional supplementation
	Abstinence counseling
	Cognitive behavioral therapy for behavior modification
	Medication
Thyroid problems	Laboratory data
	Medication
	Endocrine consult
Vitamin deficiencies	Laboratory data
	Supplementation

Table 18.2 ■ **COMMON CHRONIC DEMENTIAS**

Type of Dementia	Characteristics
Alzheimer's disease	Most common type of dementia
	Difficulty with memory is often an early clinical symptom
Vascular dementia	Second most common cause of dementia. Previously known as multi-infarct or poststroke dementia
Frontotemporal dementia (FTD)	Includes dementias such as behavioral variant FTD (bvFTD), primary progressive aphasia, Pick's disease, and progressive supranuclear palsy
Dementia with Lewy bodies	Memory loss and thinking problems. Commonly have early symptoms of sleep disturbances, well-formed visual hallucinations, and muscle rigidity or other parkinsonian movement features

(continued)

Table 18.2 ■ COMMON CHRONIC DEMENTIAS *(continued)*

Type of Dementia	Characteristics
Mixed dementia	Abnormalities linked to more than one type of dementia occur simultaneously in the brain
Wernicke–Korsakoff	Chronic memory disorder caused by severe deficiency of thiamine (vitamin B_1). The most common cause is alcohol abuse
Parkinson's disease	Common to find a progressive dementia as the disease progresses

psychiatric cause of cognitive impairment such as depression, where there is concurrent delirium, or in patients who are poorly educated or mentally handicapped. The signs and symptoms of different types of dementia overlap, which also makes diagnosing the exact type of dementia a challenge.

■ CRITERION-BASED DIAGNOSIS

The diagnosis of dementia requires a specific set of criteria. The most widely used criteria for the diagnosis of dementia are those developed by the American Psychiatric Association for the *Diagnostic and Statistical Manual of Mental Disorders (DSM)*. These criteria are recognized by the American Academy of Neurology as a clinical guideline for routine use in the diagnosis of dementia. The *DSM III* outlined a specific set of criteria for the diagnosis of dementia in general. The fourth revision of the *DSM* did not include a separate diagnosis for the dementia syndrome, but instead included criteria for the different types of dementia. Alzheimer's disease and vascular dementia are the most common causes of dementia.

To meet the *DSM-IV* criteria for Alzheimer's disease, a patient must demonstrate a memory deficit objectively on cognitive testing and have one other cognitive deficit such as aphasia (abnormal speech), executive function impairment (difficulty with planning, judgment, mental flexibility, abstraction, problem solving, etc.), agnosia (impaired recognition of people or objects), or apraxia (impaired performance of learned motor skills). Together these cognitive deficits must result in impairment in performance of daily activities. The course is characterized by gradual onset and continuing cognitive decline. These

Table 18.3 ■ SIGNS OF ALZHEIMER'S DEMENTIA COMPARED WITH NORMAL AGE-RELATED CHANGES

Task	Example of Change Seen in Alzheimer's Patient	Normal Changes With Age
Memory loss	Repeated forgetfulness, especially of recently learned information. This is one of the most common and early signs of Alzheimer's disease.	Occasionally having difficulty remembering someone's name. Missing an appointment by mistake.
Misplacing things	In addition to misplacing items, in Alzheimer's disease objects may be placed in inappropriate locations (e.g., placing car keys in the fridge).	Occasionally misplacing the car keys and finding them later.
Orientation to time and place	Losing track of the date, season, or year is common in Alzheimer's patients. They can get lost in their own neighborhood and be unable to find their way home.	Forgetting the date or day of the week and then remembering it later.
Difficulty with familiar tasks	Alzheimer's can often lead to difficulty with planning or completing everyday tasks such as preparing a familiar meal, baking a cake, or making a phone call.	Difficulty using the remote control to tape a favorite TV show.
Changes in language	Alzheimer's can lead to difficulty with following a conversation, forgetting familiar words, or substituting odd words in a sentence.	Temporarily having trouble finding the right word.
Reduced ability to make good judgment calls	Poor decision choices are common. Alzheimer's patients may dress inappropriately for the season, pay less attention to grooming, or give away large sums of money to strangers.	Occasionally making a bad judgment call.

Decreased ability with abstract thinking	Alzheimer's patients may have trouble with complex mental tasks (e.g., forgetting how to work with numbers or keeping track of monthly bills).	Having trouble with end-of-year tax returns or making an occasional arithmetic error.
Changes in mood, behavior, or personality	Rapid mood swings with no obvious triggers. Alzheimer's patients can become suspicious, fearful, or anxious.	Feeling sad or anxious on occasion.
Loss of initiative	Alzheimer's can make a person very passive, sitting in front of the TV or sleeping for long periods of time.	Needing some "down time" to mentally de-stress.
Social withdrawal	Withdrawal from hobbies, groups, or social activities is common in Alzheimer's disease, possibly because of language, comprehension, mood, and personality changes.	On occasion feeling tired of socializing.

Adapted from "Know The 10 Signs" Alzheimer's Association http://www.alz.org/national/documents/checklist_10signs.pdf

deficits must represent a decline from a previous higher level of functioning, and there must not be any other neurological disease that accounts for them. *DSM-V* has moved away from the term *dementia* in favor of using the term *neurocognitive disorders*. The *DSM-V* section on neurocognitive disorders differs significantly from the *DSM-IV*, but it has been suggested that providers may barely change how they diagnose AD and other cognitive disorders. Further discussion of these diagnostic differences is beyond the scope of this book.

As people age, there are changes in mental acuity that are natural and not related to any dementing illness. Table 18.3 outlines some additional signs and symptoms that may lead a clinician to suspect Alzheimer's disease in a presenting patient. These are highlighted against normal findings in a patient that does not have Alzheimer's.

Vascular dementia is defined by the same set of criteria that apply to Alzheimer's. In a similar fashion, the cognitive deficits must result in impairment in performance of daily activities, be gradual in onset, and represent a decline from a previous higher level of functioning. There must not be any other neurological disease that accounts for them. In addition, there may be focal neurological signs and symptoms such as weakness, or relevant cerebrovascular disease by radiographic brain imaging (CT or MRI). Other signs of vascular dementia may include

- early presence of gait disturbance
- history of unsteadiness and frequent, unprovoked falls
- early urinary frequency, urgency, and other urinary symptoms not explained by urologic disease
- pseudobulbar palsy
- personality and mood changes, abulia, depression, emotional incontinence, or other subcortical deficits including psychomotor retardation and abnormal executive functions

MIXED DEMENTIA

The brain is highly vascular. Blood vessel changes in the brain are linked to vascular dementia, which often will present along with other types of dementia, such as Alzheimer's disease. These changes may interact to cause earlier onset, faster decline of the patient, or more profound limitations.

EARLY DIAGNOSIS OF DEMENTIA

The early diagnosis of dementia can be especially difficult. The commonly used screening tests for mental dysfunction are insensitive to mild cognitive dysfunction. Diagnosis is further hampered by the fact that there is no single baseline of normal against which all patients may be compared. Some high-functioning patients may not meet the criteria for dementia despite the fact that they or their family are concerned about changes in their intellectual functioning. These patients should be evaluated over time (6 to 12 months) to be able to document a decline in mental functioning.

■ **QUESTIONS TO ASK THE PATIENT**

When possible, a close relative or friend should attend the appointments with the patient, and it should be someone who sees the patient on a consistent basis and is integral in his or her life. Questioning may be done together with both patient and relative. Sometimes, this is upsetting for the patient, or the relative is afraid to be forthright in front of the patient. In this case, have the family member come into the office for questioning first, and then bring the patient in to complete the history of present illness. Questions may include:

Has there been a change?

What kind of cognitive changes have you noticed?

Are you noticing that you are more forgetful; for example, forgetting to switch off the stove?

Has anyone else noticed any changes?

Have you experienced memory loss that disrupts your daily life?

Are you having difficulty completing familiar tasks?

Do you have difficulty with following multistep directions, planning, or problem solving?

Have you been confused with time or place?

Are you having any new problems with words in speaking or writing?

Are you feeling less social?

How is your mood?

■ IMPORTANT LABS

When assessing a patient for dementia, it is necessary to run diagnostic testing to rule out readily treatable metabolic and structural causes. Generally, the laboratory tests should include a complete blood count, serum electrolytes including calcium, glucose, and blood urea nitrogen (BUN), liver function tests, thyroid stimulating hormone level, serum B_{12} level, and methylmelonic acid level.

■ IMPORTANT IMAGING

Imaging studies help identify possible treatable conditions such as tumors, subdural hematomas, hydrocephalus, and strokes. Relative to the natural incidence of dementia, these conditions are reasonably uncommon, but the testing is straightforward, and some of these conditions are treatable.

■ ADDITIONAL TESTING

In the office, testing of mental status can be done using screening tools such as the Mini-Mental State Exam, 6CIT, or the MoCA, which result in numeric scores that can then be tracked over time (See Chapter 2 for a lengthier discussion on mental status testing.) Although not always required, neuropsychological testing may be helpful in cases where the clinical diagnosis of dementia is borderline or decisions need to be made about the patient's competency, job, or personal affairs. In addition, it may help to separate out dementia from depression.

■ DEMENTIA RISK, PREVENTION, AND TREATMENT

Age, gender, and genetics are predetermined risk factors for dementia, over which the patient has no control. However, we know that there are some modifiable factors. In general, it can be said that "What is good for your heart is good for your head." Smoking status, cardiovascular risk, sleep, exercise, and diet can help prevent the onset and severity of the disease.

EXERCISE

Longitudinal studies have found that consistent exercise throughout a person's life plays a significant role in reducing the risk of developing dementia. When compared with not smoking, low body weight, healthy diet, and low alcohol intake, aerobic exercise had the single biggest influence on the incidence and prognosis of dementia. Although not well understood, modest aerobic exercise, in as little as 6 months to 1 year, has been shown to increase brain volumes, specifically in the prefrontal cortex and hippocampus. Both of these regions deteriorate and shrink as we get older. The prefrontal cortex is responsible for higher level cognitive functions, and the hippocampus is involved in memory formation, which is an integral part of the dementing illnesses.

NUTRITION

Reversible dementias, such as B_{12} deficiency and folate deficiencies, may be managed with good nutrition and supplementation. Alcoholic dementia is due both to the direct neurotoxic effects of the alcohol and to the patient's poor nutritional status. This may be at least partially reversible with abstinence and good nutrition.

Although there has been no direct link between fat intake and the risk of dementia, current thinking links a heart-healthy diet with one that will also protect the brain. This would include a diet that is rich in fruits and vegetables, whole grains, and healthy fats such as olive or nut oils. This is particularly true for vascular or multi-infarct dementias. In all types of dementia, excellent nutrition may help maximize the patient's physical well-being and improve the quality of life.

SLEEP

Sleep is important in the learning and memory systems of the brain. Recent research has shown that sleep allows for the clearing of toxic substances from the brain. It does this through the glymphatic system, which is the brain's equivalent of the lymphatic system. Many of the dementia subgroups, such as Alzheimer's disease, are characterized by the build-up of damaged proteins in the brain. It may be postulated that a defective glymphatic system may contribute to such diseases, but definitive cause and effect has not yet been shown. There is mounting evidence that sleep may contribute to the restoration of brain cell function and may have protective effects. In patients with dementia, disrupted sleep–wake cycles are common. Managing insomnia becomes an important part of managing the disease.

MEDICATION

The U.S. Food and Drug Administration (FDA) has approved two types of medications to treat the cognitive symptoms (memory loss, confusion, and problems with thinking and reasoning) of Alzheimer's disease, namely cholinesterase inhibitors (Aricept, Exelon, Razadyne, Cognex) and Memantine (Namenda).

Diplopia

Double vision, also known as diplopia, may be a patient's presenting symptom, or it may be elicited during the course of an eye examination. Care should be taken to ensure that the patient is describing true double vision and not just blurry vision or metamorphopsia, in which objects appear misshapen. Diplopia can be the first manifestation of many systemic disorders, especially muscular or neurological processes. An accurate, clear description of the symptoms (e.g., constant or intermittent; variable or unchanging; at near or at far; with one eye [monocular] or with both eyes [binocular]; horizontal, vertical, or oblique) is critical to appropriate diagnosis and management.

The seemingly simple process of seeing a single clear image depends on the orchestration of multiple areas of the vision system (Figure 19.1). They all need to work together seamlessly:

- The cornea is the clear window into the eye. It does most of the focusing of incoming light.
- The lens is behind the pupil. It also helps focus light onto the retina.
- Muscles of the eye—extraocular muscles—rotate the eye.
- Nerves carry visual information from the eyes to the brain.
- Several areas of the brain process visual information from the eyes.

Problems with any part of the vision system can lead to double vision.

Monocular diplopia is when the patient sees double with only one eye open. Commonly in monocular diplopia, the second image is seen as a ghost. Monocular diplopia results from a refractive error of the eye, meaning that in all cases of monocular

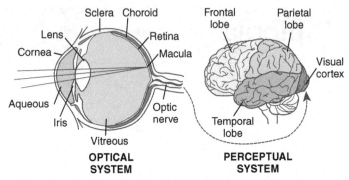

Figure 19.1 ◼ Schematic diagram of the visual system

diplopia, the defect is anterior to the retina. These include abnormal ocular media, corneal distortion or scarring, multiple openings in the iris, cataract or subluxation of the natural lens or pseudophakic lens implant, vitreous abnormalities, and retinal conditions.

Binocular diplopia is when the patient sees double only when both eyes are open. Covering either eye resolves the double vision. Binocular diplopia is a result of breakdown in the binocular visual system. This breakdown may be a result of an inability to maintain synchronicity in muscle movements of the eye when looking at an object, resulting in the visual object not being projected onto the two retinas in the same way. Rarely, binocular visual fusion of an image cannot occur because of dissimilar image size, which can occur following refractive surgery (e.g., LASIK) or after a cataract is replaced by an intraocular lens. The distortion of one image may be interpreted as diplopia by the patient; however, the same object does not appear to be in two places but rather appears differently with each eye.

◼ **NERVE PALSIES**

There are six muscles that control movement of the eye. These six muscles are innervated by three cranial nerves (CN): CN III, IV, and VI. The primary presenting symptoms when there is damage to these nerves is diplopia as the eye muscle is not innervated correctly, causing weakness. If a muscle in one eye is weak, that eye cannot move smoothly in concert with the other healthy eye.

Gazing in directions controlled by the weak muscle causes double vision. The orientation of the diplopia will depend on which cranial nerve is affected. For a more in-depth discussion on palsies of the CN III, IV, and VI, please refer to Chapter 4.

A cranial nerve palsy may be complete or partial, affecting the structures served by this nerve either completely or partially. In the case of a cranial nerve that has multiple functions, such as CN III, it is possible for a palsy to affect all of the various functions or only some of the functions of that nerve.

THIRD NERVE PALSY

CN III plays a major role in eye movement. It innervates four of the six extraocular eye muscles. In addition, it innervates muscles that control the shape of the lens and the size of the pupils (the constrictor pupillae and ciliary muscle).

Damage to CN III affecting the extraocular muscles will result in the patient being unable to focus both eyes on the same object, resulting in double vision.

FOURTH NERVE PALSY

The trochlear nerve, CN IV, is the smallest of the cranial nerves and innervates only a single muscle, the superior oblique muscle. When the superior oblique muscle stops functioning, the inferior oblique extorts and slightly elevates the eye. This lack of concordance between the eyes results in the image projected onto different areas of the right and left retinas, resulting in two distinct images being seen. Tilting the head away from the dysfunctional side may improve the patient's vision by obliging the opposite site to intort and thereby compensating.

A fourth nerve palsy can be very difficult to detect; observing the downward gaze when the eye is adducted may be the most sensitive test.

SIXTH NERVE PALSY

The abducens nerve, CN VI, like its counterpart CN IV, innervates only one muscle, the lateral rectus muscle. It is a somatic motor nerve with the sole function of moving the eye laterally away from midline. A patient with a sixth nerve palsy will have double vision when looking at an object to the same side as the lesion, but when looking away from the lesion, the double vision will resolve.

Cranial nerve palsies may be present from birth or acquired later in life as a result of trauma, infection, tumor, or vascular disease. The vascular diseases that most commonly affect the eye include diabetes, hypertension, strokes, and aneurysms.

■ TESTING FOR DIPLOPIA

BINOCULAR DIPLOPIA

When testing for double vision, have the patient look in all four quadrants of his or her visual field. This is done by having the patient follow your finger as you draw a box or an "H" in the air in front of the patient. If there is an extraocular eye movement (EOM) deficiency, it may only show up in one of the quadrants. Explain to the patient that he or she should report double vision. Also note whether the double vision is horizontal (side-by-side images) or vertical (images lying one on top of another). The matter of horizontal or vertical double vision is an important one. In general, vertical double vision comes from a central source (cerebellar), but may also be seen in fourth nerve palsy. Horizontal double vision most commonly comes from a peripheral source, such as misalignment of the eyes secondary to asynchronous eye movements. From a practical perspective, eye tracking should be done prior to examination of the internal structure of the eye, both for the comfort of the patient (after a bright light has been shone in the patient's eye) and for the best testing outcome.

As you evaluate the patient for double vision, check the alignment of the eyes. They should at all times be aligned with each other. In certain people, for example patients of East Asian descent, it may be hard to objectively make that call. In such cases, use a flashlight to shine light across the eyes so that a reflection is seen on the iris of both eyes; the location of the reflection on the iris should be aligned. Subtle differences in eye alignment may be seen clearly using this technique.

MULTIPLE SCLEROSIS

Multiple sclerosis (MS) is an autoimmune disease that causes damage to the myelin sheath of nerve cells in the central nervous system (brain, optic nerve, and spinal cord). Vision problems are common in MS and may be the first presenting sign. These include optic neuritis, nystagmus, and diplopia.

Diplopia is typically due to either a sixth nerve palsy secondary to an ocular motor cranial neuropathy or to internuclear ophthalmoplegia (INO). Third and fourth cranial neuropathies are uncommon in MS. INO is a specific gaze abnormality where there is impaired horizontal eye movement. There is an adduction deficit of the affected eye, with horizontal gaze nystagmus in the contralateral abducting eye. This is a very localizing finding resulting from a lesion in the medial longitudinal fasciculus (MLF) in the dorsomedial brainstem tegmentum of either the pons or the midbrain. A high level of suspicion for MS should be had in a young patient presenting with bilateral INO.

Diplopia in MS usually resolves without treatment. Symptoms of double vision may increase with fatigue and, therefore, resting the eyes may help improve symptoms. In some cases, a brief course of corticosteroids is warranted. Patching one eye can be useful when specific tasks need to be accomplished, such as driving, but is not recommended for long periods of time.

MYESTHENIA GRAVIS

Myesthenia gravis (MG) is a disorder of neuromuscular transmission characterized by weakness and fatigability of skeletal muscles. This is an acquired autoimmune disease in which there is a reduced number of acetylcholine receptors (AChRs) at the postsynaptic muscle membrane due to anti-AChR antibodies.

Most patients with MG develop ophthalmologic manifestations of the disease. Extraocular muscle involvement does not follow a specific pattern. MG may present as an isolated muscle palsy, total external ophthalmoplegia, or somewhere in between. Any acquired disturbance in ocular motor functioning, with or without ptosis but with normally reacting pupils, should raise suspicion for MG.

GRAVES'S DISEASE

Graves's disease is an autoimmune condition in which immune cells attack the thyroid gland and cause a hypermetabolic state. There is an associated condition known as Graves's eye disease, where the eye muscle and connective tissue become the targets of autoimmune attack. Most probably this occurs because these tissues contain proteins that appear similar to the immune system, for example, those of the thyroid gland. In severe cases of Graves's eye disease, the inflammation of the muscles causes muscular swelling and stiffness. This interferes with movement of the eyes, which subsequently can cause double vision.

The principal treatment for Graves's eye disease involves treatment of the underlying thyroid condition. This includes medications to suppress the production of hormone by the thyroid gland, radioactive iodine ablation to eliminate hormone-producing cells, and/or surgery to remove the thyroid tissue. The eye disease must be closely monitored by an ophthalmologist as it often continues to progress even after the underlying thyroid condition has been treated. Additional ophthalmologic intervention such as short-term steroids, radiation, or surgical intervention may be needed to preserve sight.

MILLER FISHER SYNDROME

Miller Fisher syndrome (MFS) is a rare variant of Guillain-Barré syndrome (GBS), observed in less than 5% of all cases. MFS is characterized by the triad of areflexia, ataxia, and ophthalmoplegia. In patients with MFS, the first nerve groups to be affected by paralysis are those in the head. As a result, eye movement abnormalities are a prominent feature in MFS. Difficulty controlling eye muscles affects conjugate gaze and results in diplopia. In contrast, paralysis typically begins in the legs and rarely involves the eyes in other more common variants of GBS.

Generally, MFS is self-limiting, but more severe cases may be treated with intravenous immunoglobulin (IVIg) or plasmaphoresis. Recovery can be expected to begin within 2 to 4 weeks and complete resolution of symptoms occurs typically within 6 months. Most patients make a full recovery with no residual neurological deficits.

DIABETES

Uncontrolled diabetes can lead to nerve infarction and subsequent palsy. This is due to damage to the small blood vessels that feed the nerve and is part of the diabetic peripheral neuropathy syndrome. Infarction of CN III with a resultant third nerve palsy is the most common, but CN IV and CN VI may also be affected in a similar manner.

CENTRAL NERVOUS SYSTEM LESIONS

Skew deviation is a prenuclear vertical misalignment that results from brainstem or cerebellar lesions. Many different causes for double vision originate in the brain. They include strokes; aneurysms; increased pressure inside the brain from trauma, bleeding, or infection; brain tumors; or migraine headaches.

MONOCULAR DIPLOPIA

Monocular diplopia is caused by refractive errors of the eye. Monocular diplopia is always a result of defects in the eye from the retina forward; there is no cause of monocular diplopia farther back than the retina.

Common causes of monocular diplopia are corneal and lens problems. Problems with the cornea often cause double vision in one eye only. Covering the affected eye makes the double vision go away. The abnormal surface of the eye distorts incoming light, causing double vision. There are a number of things that may cause damage to the cornea, including infections of the cornea (herpes zoster or shingles), corneal scars, or dryness of the cornea. Cataracts are the most common problem with the lens that causes double vision. If cataracts are present in both eyes, images from both eyes will be distorted. Cataracts are often correctable with minor surgery.

When considering the patient with diplopia it is of paramount importance that some diagnoses are not missed. These include the following: If all eye defects have been ruled out, it is possible that the report of double vision by a patient using a single eye is a marker of embellishment of the exam. Standard of care would require that such eye defects be ruled out, after which the value of the patient's report may come into question.

- Tumor of orbit
- Tumor along cranial nerve pathway
- Increased intracranial pressure resulting in bilateral abducens palsy
- Aneurysm of intracranial carotid artery
- Carotid cavernous fistula: Angiography may be required to confirm the presence of a low-flow fistula
- A blow-out fracture requires imaging of the orbital floor
- Enlarged muscles from thyroid ophthalmopathy help explain a vertical diplopia
- Disease of sinuses (e.g., infection, tumor) or bony disorders (e.g., dysostoses, encephalocele) can account for displacement of the eye

■ QUESTIONS TO ASK THE PATIENT

Is this double vision constant or intermittent?

Is it more pronounced at near or at far?

Is this change in vision associated with pain?

Have you experienced a trauma such as being hit on the head or fallen?

Is the double vision worse at the end of the day or when you're tired?

Have you had any other symptoms besides double vision?

Are the two objects side by side, or is one on top of the other? Or are they slightly diagonal?

Are both images clear but simply unaligned with each other? Or is one image blurry and the other clear?

Cover one eye, then uncover it and cover the other. Does covering either eye make the double vision go away?

Tilt your head to the right, then to the left. Do any of these positions improve the double vision, or make it worse?

■ IMPORTANT LABS

Laboratory studies may be performed on the basis of suspected etiology of the diplopia or to rule out a given cause.

■ IMPORTANT IMAGING

Order a CT scan or MRI (with contrast) of the skull and orbits to rule out intracranial masses or other pathologic processes. Traditional guidelines for imaging patients with new-onset diplopia include imaging all patients younger than 50 years with other neurological findings, with a progressive course of diplopia, or with a history of cancer. For patients older than 50 years, imaging is not always necessary during the initial evaluation.

■ TREATMENT

With double vision, the most important step is to identify and treat the underlying cause. If double vision cannot be reversed or controlled by controlling the underlying etiology, treatments can help people live with double vision. Sometimes this requires wearing an eye patch or special prism glasses to minimize the effect of double vision.

Gait Disturbance 20

Gait disorders are walking patterns that deviate uncontrollably from the norm, and are usually due to diseases or injuries to the brain, spinal cord, legs, feet, or inner ear. These changes in gait can be temporary or chronic. When chronic, a patient may require intensive, ongoing treatment. Certain disease processes commonly cause a gait disturbance, such as multiple sclerosis and Parkinson's disease. Other diseases are not typically thought of as associated with gait change such as liver disease or pernicious anemia.

■ CLINICAL APPROACH

Examination of the patient with a gait disorder starts with watching the patient walk. The act of walking involves numerous systems, and a change in any one of these systems may cause a walking problem. The neurological examination for a gait disturbance needs to include tests of strength, muscle tone, coordination, proprioception, the vestibular system, and cortical function including the frontal lobes. A more in-depth discussion on the mechanics of gait and balance testing, as well as classification of gaits, are outlined in Chapter 10.

Muscle weakness, muscle tightness, and balance problems are common causes of gait disturbance. Muscle weakness can cause problems such as foot drop (tibialis anterior, weakness), a Trendelenburg gait, or circumduction (swinging leg out to the side). Spasticity (muscle tightness) can also interfere with gait. Balance problems typically result in an ataxic gate, characterized by a swaying, drunken appearance.

The most common gait disturbances and their possible etiologies are summarized in Table 20.1.

Table 20.1 ■ **COMMON GAIT DISTURBANCES AND POSSIBLE ETIOLOGIES**

Gait	Common Presenting Illness
Ataxic gait	■ Multiple sclerosis ■ Advanced diabetes ■ Alcohol intoxication ■ Brain injury ■ Acute cerebellar ataxia
Antalgic gait	■ Trauma ■ Osteoarthritis
Hemiplegic gait	■ Stroke
Propulsive gait	■ Parkinson's disease ■ Carbon monoxide poisoning ■ Medication (e.g., haloperidol [Haldol])
Scissors gait	■ Spastic cerebral palsy
Spastic gait	■ Brain lesions including abscesses, tumors and demyelinating diseases ■ Multiple sclerosis ■ Brain trauma ■ Stroke ■ Cerebral palsy ■ Cervical spondylosis or degenerative disc disease with myelopathy ■ Liver failure ■ Pernicious anemia ■ Spinal cord lesion including tumors, demyelinating disease or the presence of a syrinx
Steppage gait	■ Foot drop due to compression of the L4 nerve root ■ Tibialis anterior weakness ■ Multiple sclerosis
Waddling gait	■ Congenital hip dysplasia ■ Myopathies ■ Spinal muscle atrophy

Changes in gait, such as slower walking or a more variable stride and rhythm, may be early signs of neurocognitive disorders before other clinical signs are present or a more formal diagnosis is made. In one study of Alzheimer's disease, patients with decreased cadence, speed, and stride length showed larger declines in overall cognition, memory, and executive function.

PARKINSON'S DISEASE

Parkinson's disease (PD) is a chronic and progressive neurological disorder affecting neurons in the substantia nigra, a dopamine-producing area of the brain. Dopamine is involved in controlling movement and coordination. As PD progresses, the amount of dopamine produced in the brain decreases, leaving a person unable to control movement normally. This results in tremor, rigidity, slowness, and postural instability. A disturbed gait is a common and debilitating symptom, and one that represents a major therapeutic challenge. A parkinsonian gait encompasses three components: a hypokinetic gait, freezing of gait, and a festination (further explanation of these gaits may be found in Chapter 10). These symptoms may not be severe early in the course of PD, but they progress with time in a majority of the cases and represent a heavier burden later in the course of the disease.

Patients with severe gait disturbances are prone to falls, which increases their risk of mortality and morbidity. Most falls are unrelated to external factors, such as slipping, but rather are dependent upon inherent deficits of balance control. Falls occur mainly during posture changes or when multitasking is required where there are both cognitive and motor demands on the patient.

Gait disturbances respond best to dopaminergic treatments in the early phase of the disease; consequently, rehabilitation appears to be the most effective approach to gait changes in the Parkinsonian patient.

ALZHEIMER'S DISEASE

Gait disorders are common in patients with Alzheimer's disease (AD). Patients with mild dementia exhibit a cautious gait that is expressed as impaired static balance, slow gait speed, and short stride length. Frontal gait disorder is the most common gait disturbance in patients with moderate to severe AD. Frontal gait is characterized by prominent disequilibrium, short steps, shuffling, and start and turn hesitation. Unsteadiness of gait increases with progression of AD and may be associated with progressive rigidity and asynchrony of gait as the dementia increases in severity. Frontal gait is not unique to AD and may be seen in patients with multiple lacunar infarcts, Binswanger disease, frontal lobe tumor, and hydrocephalus.

MULTIPLE SCLEROSIS

Multiple sclerosis (MS) is a disease that invariably affects the patient's ability to walk. This is related to several factors including muscle weakness, spasticity, sensory ataxia, and fatigue.

Muscle weakness most commonly presents first as a foot drop resulting in circumduction of the foot on the affected side. In addition, in later stages of the disease, muscle weakness may cause quadriceps weakness, seen as knee hyperextension, trunk flexion, or increased lumbar lordosis, and weakness through the hip abductors, resulting in a Trendelenburg gait with a lean to the weak side. Weakness may be mitigated in part with physical therapy and assistive devices, including braces, canes, or walkers.

Spasticity is a common finding in MS and can significantly interfere with gait. Stretching exercises and antispasticity medications such as baclofen or tizanidine are first line treatment for these symptoms. Owing to difficulty with balance and sensory deficits in their feet, ataxia is common. Fatigue augments gait disturbances for MS patients and makes compensation for their sensory ataxia more of a challenge.

Ampyra (dalfampridine) is currently the only FDA drug on the market to improve gait speed in MS. It can be very helpful; however, it does not help every MS patient. Clinical trials have shown improvement in walking speed in 25% of patients in all forms of MS.

DIABETES

Nerve damage results from poorly managed and chronically high levels of blood sugar. This causes neuropathy, with peripheral sensory neuropathy being the most common form of diabetic neuropathy. Diabetic peripheral neuropathy tends to decrease walking speed and cause patients to widen their stance changes gait, with patients tending to walk more slowly and with a wider stance than those without neuropathy.

Glucose dysmetabolism is the primary cause of diabetic neuropathy. Elevated blood sugars cause irritation, damage, and ultimately nerve death. Small nerve fibers are particularly susceptible to this type of damage. Small nerve fiber damage results in burning pain, paresthesias, and electric shock sensations, and may ultimately result in complete loss of sensation. Neuropathic changes in the diabetic patient present in a distal-to-proximal gradient, resulting in a stocking distribution effect that affects the feet first and then systematically progresses up the lower limbs. Rarely does small fiber neuropathy follow a non–length dependent distribution. There appears to be a direct correlation between glucose impairment and the extent of nerve damage. Owing to loss of protective sensation, patients with sensory loss in the lower extremities have a heightened risk of foot complications such as foot ulcers, infection, and gangrene. They are also more prone to callus formation, edema, and stress fractures. This may impair daily living activities and increase the risk of falls and fractures.

Damage to large nerve fibers occurs in a process not unlike that of small nerve fiber damage. Loss of proprioception and coordination due to large nerve fiber damage challenges gait and balance further.

Motor neuropathy can accompany sensory loss, and presents as loss of deep tendon reflexes (patellar and Achilles) and muscle weakness. Foot dorsiflexion is compromised owing to damage of the peroneal nerve, resulting in foot drop and toe drag. Logically, this is known as diabetic foot drop. Ankle-foot orthosis (AFO) may be used to help alleviate the problem of diabetic foot drop.

■ QUESTIONS TO ASK THE PATIENT

When did this problem with walking begin?

Did this change in gait happen suddenly or gradually?

When does it occur?

Has it become worse over time?

Is there pain?

Are there any other concurrent symptoms?

Have others noticed this change in gait?

■ IMPORTANT LABS

If drug or toxin exposure is suspected then the relevant labs should be run. For patients with a suspicion of diabetes or metabolic syndrome, a hemoglobin A1C and lipid panel can be checked.

■ IMPORTANT IMAGING

There is no standard imaging that is required for the assessment of a gait disturbance unless a central nervous system lesion, increased intracranial pressure, or head trauma is suspected. In those cases, MRI would be the imaging of choice to rule out lesion or increased intracranial pressure and CT and/or MRI for an acute head trauma.

■ TREATMENT

Treating the cause of the gait disturbance often leads to improvment in the gait. For example, gait changes due to leg injury will improve as the leg heals, and changes in gait due to increased intracranial pressure resolve as the intracranial pressure resolves.

PHYSICAL THERAPY

Most gait problems, either acute or chronic, can be helped to some extent by physical therapy. Therapy will strengthen core muscles and improve balance, which in turn will reduce the risk of falls and other injuries. Physical therapy centers around the right therapy for the right diagnosis. In sending a patient to physical therapy without a clear diagnosis of the problem, it is imperative to allow the physical therapist the opportunity to tailor the therapy regimen to meet the patient's needs and goals.

ASSISTIVE DEVICES AND ORTHODICS

Patients with weakness and an unbalanced gait may benefit from the use of assistive devices such as braces, canes, or walkers.

SPASTICITY

Stretching exercises and antispasticity medications such as baclofen or tizanidine are the mainstays of treatment for this symptom.

Headache

Headaches present as a common complaint in both the primary care physician's and the neurologist's office. Headaches can be completely disabling and can significantly interfere with the patient's activities of daily living. The challenge with headaches is separating out the benign from those that are more serious, as frequently, the initial presenting symptoms are similar. Here, we focus on primary headache syndromes that are both common and typically benign in nature. Common primary causes of headache are presented in Table 21.1 and are discussed here. Secondary headache syndromes are briefly referred to with reference to headache emergencies in Table 21.2, but full discussion is beyond the scope of this book.

■ CLINICAL APPROACHES TO HEADACHES AND HEAD PAIN

Primary headache syndromes have no additional underlying pathology. When a new-onset headache presents, it is paramount to rule out all serious pathology before ascribing the headache to a benign cause. Although primary headaches are considered benign in nature, they can be debilitating for the patient and significantly impact the functionality and quality of life. Correct diagnosis of headache type allows for directed treatment choice.

MIGRAINES

Migraines are among the most common causes of headaches. The International Headache Society diagnoses a migraine by the nature of its pain and number of attacks. Typical characteristics of

Table 21.1 ■ COMMON PRIMARY CAUSES OF HEADACHES AND THEIR PRESENTING SYMPTOMS

Headache	Onset and Duration	Distinctive Quality	Comments
Medication overuse headache	Continuous	May be suspected whenever increasing amounts of medication are required to keep symptoms at bay	Treatment may be challenging during the washout period. There is no evidence that shows tapering down helps the process.
Migraine	Acute onset >4 hr	Commonly unilateral and throbbing in quality. Photophobia, phonophobia, nausea, and vomiting	Common onset at puberty. For women, may change in quality or frequency in menopause.
Cluster headaches	5–15 min	Sharp stabbing sensation. Generally unilateral in the frontal and temporal regions. Watery eye and runny nose on affected side	Although short in duration, these headaches can be blindingly intense and, therefore, quite disabling.
Tension headaches	>4 hr	Continuous banding-type pain	Mild-to-moderate, vise-like pressure. The pain is frequently bilateral, and on occasion may be severe.
Exertional headaches	Acute	Onset with exertion	Throbbing, bilateral pain that becomes severe very quickly after a strenuous activity.
Trigeminal neuralgia	A few seconds at a time	Episodic attacks of excruciating, lightning-like pain on one side of the face	Generally idiopathic, although may be the result of a previous viral infection or trauma.

Table 21.2 ■ CANNOT-MISS CAUSES OF HEADACHES AND THEIR ASSOCIATED SYMPTOMS

Headache	Associated Symptoms	Distinctive Quality	Comments
Medication/Toxin			
Carbon monoxide poisoning	Lightheadedness, confusion, vertigo, and flu-like symptoms	Suspicion of poisoning by the patient's history of present illness	Toxic to the central nervous system
Intracranial			
Subarachnoid hemorrhage	Photophobia	Thunderclap headache	Although the thunderclap headache is most typically associated with a subarachnoid hemorrhage, there may be other etiologies
	Phonophobia		
	Nausea and vomiting		
Pituitary apoplexy	Associated with nausea and vomiting and visual field defect or diplopia	Acute-onset headache located behind the eyes or around the temples	Occasionally, the presence of blood leads to meningeal irritation, causing nuchal rigidity, photophobia, as well as a decreased level of consciousness
Vascular			
Intracranial bleed	Photophobia	Various, but often a dull generalized pain	These headaches may be seen in trauma, but also may be a function of chronic intracranial bleeding, especially if a patient has been on anticoagulants or antiplatelet agents including the use of high doses of nonsteroidal anti-inflammatory drugs (NSAIDs)

(continued)

Table 21.2 ■ CANNOT-MISS CAUSES OF HEADACHES AND THEIR ASSOCIATED SYMPTOMS (*continued*)

Headache	Associated Symptoms	Distinctive Quality	Comments
Intracranial bleed (*continued*)	Phonophobia		
	Nausea and vomiting		
	Change in mentation (occurs later)		
Temporal arteritis	Reduced visual acuity, acute visual loss diplopia, acute tinnitus	Tenderness and sensitivity on the scalp	Emergent to prevent permanent vision loss. More common in women, the mean age of onset is >55 years. Strong association with polymyalgia rheumatica
	Elevated erythrocyte sedimentation rate (ESR)		
Arterial dissection	Horner's syndrome	Headache in the setting of acute visual changes	May be either spontaneous or traumatic in origin
			70% of patients with carotid arterial dissection are between the ages of 35 and 50

Venous sinus thrombosis	Abnormal vision, any of the symptoms of stroke such as weakness of the face and limbs on one side of the body, and seizures		Although it may occur in all age groups, it is most common women in their thirties
Intracranial Pressure			
Idiopathic intracranial hypertension (pseudotumor ceribri)	Nausea and vomiting, as well as pulsatile tinnitus, double vision, and other visual symptoms	Pain increases with lying supine or bending forward	Most commonly seen in young overweight women. May resolve with weight loss
Cerebral spinal fluid (CSF) leak (intracranial hypotension)		Orthostatic headache (i.e., one that occurs or worsens with upright posture)	Pain is decreased with lying supine and increased with standing
Meningitis, infection, or abscess	Nuchal rigidity		

(continued)

Table 21.2 ■ CANNOT-MISS CAUSES OF HEADACHES AND THEIR ASSOCIATED SYMPTOMS (*continued*)

Headache	Associated Symptoms	Distinctive Quality	Comments
Tumor	May have no other symptoms, but typically the associated symptoms will vary with the location of the tumor		Headache-producing tumors are generally large enough to cause mass effect
Colloidal cyst of the third ventricle	Headache, nausea, or other signs of increased intracranial hypertension	Pain increases with lying supine or bending forward. It is also exacerbated by laughing, coughing, jugular venous compression, and Valsalva maneuver	Causes obstructive hypertension and increased intracranial pressure. Pain is resistant to treatment with analgesic agents.

the migrainous headache are unilateral location, pulsating quality, moderate or severe intensity, aggravation by routine physical activity, and association with nausea and/or photophobia and phonophobia. For diagnosis, at least five episodes are required where, if untreated, the pain would last from 4 to 72 hours.

It is common for the patient to experience symptoms in addition to head pain including nausea and vomiting, or sensitivity to both light and sound. For the provider, photophobia, phonophobia, and nausea are comforting marks of a migrainous headache. Although these are the common migrainous symptoms, a migraine may exist with all, some, or none of them. In addition, the presence of these symptoms does not preclude a nonmigrainous etiology.

As many as 30% of migraneurs can predict the onset of a migraine because it is preceded by an aura. The aura usually precedes but sometimes accompanies the head pain, and is primarily characterized by focal neurological symptoms. This aura may be any number of symptoms, the most typical being visual disturbances such as scintillations, flashing lights, zig-zag lines, a temporary loss of vision, or changes in smell.

It is common for migraines to have a triggering factor. The most common triggers include dietary-related factors such as fasting or tyrosine-rich foods; environmental factors, such as changes in barometric pressure and bright or flashing lights; and physical factors including irregular sleep patterns, food, hormones, and stress. It is very common for tyrosine-rich food substances to trigger migraines; foods that are tyrosine-rich include red wine, aged cheese, chocolate, and citrus fruits.

Migraines are more common in women than in men, and are indiscriminate to age or race.

CLUSTER HEADACHE

Cluster headaches, also known as suicide headaches, are excruciating headaches with a poorly understood etiology, although they are thought to be neurovascular in nature. The quality of pain is described as excruciating, stabbing, or sharp, unlike the throbbing pain experienced in migraines.

According to the diagnostic criteria developed by the International Headache Society (IHS), cluster headaches are classified as attacks of severe or very severe, strictly unilateral pain (orbital, supraorbital, or temporal) that last 15 minutes to 3 hours and occur from once every other day to eight times a day. Cluster headaches present with clear periodicity, as a grouping (or cluster) over a period of several weeks described as a cluster period. The patient may experience several of these cluster periods per year.

Cluster headaches are associated with tearing of the eye, miosis and ptosis on the affected side, rhinorrhea, nasal congestion, and facial sweating. The headaches occur particularly during sleep or early morning hours, and are strongly associated with the onset of rapid eye movement (REM) sleep.

Cluster headaches may be episodic, in which each cluster phase is separated by a cluster-free interval of 1 month or longer. Chronic cluster headaches occur without remission, or the cluster-free interval is shorter than 1 month.

In relation to migraines, their occurrence is relatively uncommon, and unlike migraines they occur more frequently in men than in women.

Part of treatment of cluster headaches is educating the patient to avoid known triggers. Alcohol, tobacco, and high altitudes are known precipitants. Other triggers are similar to those listed in Table 21.4 for migraines.

TENSION HEADACHES

A tension-type headache is the most common type of primary headache, accounting for nearly 90% of all headaches. The pain from a tension headache tends to radiate around the head in a generalized fashion, behind the eyes and into the neck.

The quality of pain experienced in a tension-type headache is described as a mild-to-moderate, vise-like pressure. The pain is frequently bilateral and on occasion may be severe. Typically symptoms may last 4 to 6 hours, but there is no true standard as pain can last for hours to months and even years and may be intermittent or chronic.

EXERTIONAL HEADACHES

Primary exertional headaches are described as throbbing, bilateral pain that occurs after exertion. The onset of these headaches is acute after a strenuous activity such as weight lifting, running, or sexual intercourse. Activities that increase intracranial pressure such as coughing, sneezing or straining with bowel movements may also trigger these headaches.

MEDICATION OVERUSE HEADACHES/REBOUND HEADACHES

Rebound headaches or medication overuse headaches are secondary to the excessive use of medication. They are typically daily headaches that are relieved by the use of the offending medication. This group of headaches typically coexist with another headache condition, which is the reason the patient was using the medication in the first place. They are notoriously difficult to break and almost always involve some discomfort on the part of the patient, so patient buy-in is essential. A slow tapering off the medication in certain patients may be helpful, but there is no guarantee that this will ameliorate the patient's symptoms.

THUNDERCLAP HEADACHE

Thunderclap headache refers to an acute, severe, and explosive headache, which presents as unexpectedly as a "clap of thunder." It is a presenting symptom of various sinister underlying causes including subarachnoid hemorrhage, cerebral venous sinus thrombosis, pituitary apoplexy, spontaneous intracranial hypotension, hypertensive encephalopathy, and an idiopathic benign recurrent headache syndrome. There are no presenting symptoms that can reliably distinguish between subarachnoid hemorrhage and benign thunderclap headache, and therefore, all patients should receive a complete workup. It cannot be emphasized enough that diagnosis of an idiopathic thunderclap headache is a diagnosis of exclusion.

All patients who present with a thunderclap headache require emergent CT imaging. If the CT imaging is negative, equivocal, or technically inadequate, a lumbar puncture is indicated.

■ QUESTIONS TO ASK THE PATIENT

When was your first headache (ever in your life), and what was it like?

When did this headache start, and is it different from those that you have had before?

Where is the pain? (Use one finger to point to the location where it is worst.)

Does the pain move or generalize?

Is the pain continuous or intermittent?

How long does the headache last?

Use some words to describe the pain (sharp, shooting, stabbing, dull, throbbing, pressing, squeezing, etc.).

How bad is the pain at its worst and at its best?

Does the pain change during the day?

Is there a pattern associated with the pain (menstrual cycle, weather, mornings)?

Are there any associated symptoms (nausea and vomiting, photophobia, phonophobia)?

What makes the headache better or worse?

Do you have a family history of headaches, seizures, strokes, aneurysms?

■ USEFUL LABORATORY TESTS

A number of laboratory studies may be run depending on the suspected etiology of the headache. Most commonly, chemistries include a complete metabolic panel and complete blood count with differential B_{12} and methylmelonic acid. Thyroid function tests (TSH and free T4) may prove useful, especially if a patient has a hyperthyroid syndrome. Erythrocyte sedimentation rate (ESR) is important when ruling out suspected temporal arteritis. ESR values greater than 40 should raise suspicion and require further investigation.

■ IMAGING

Screening patients with isolated, nontraumatic headache by means of CT or MRI is generally not required. In certain circumstances, however, imaging the patient may be prudent. Table 21.3 outlines the most common useful imaging studies for headache workup.

A CT scan is useful for ruling out acute intracranial hemorrhages, and as such is the imaging of choice for new and acute headaches. CT imaging for subarachnoid hemorrhage shows a

Table 21.3 ■ MOST COMMON OR USEFUL IMAGING STUDIES FOR HEADACHES WORKUP

Headache Type	Suggested Imaging
Chronic headache with no new features	None recommended
Chronic headache with new neurological findings	MRI
Sudden-onset "thunderclap" headache	CT without contrast
Sudden onset unilateral headache (suspicion of carotid dissection)	CT without contrast or MRI with and without contrast
Suspected temporal arteritis. New headache in patients older than age 60, sedimentation rate higher than 55, temporal tenderness	MRI without contrast
Suspected complication of an ear infection, sinusitis, or mastoiditis	MRI with and without contrast

sensitivity of 100% and 98%, respectively, within the first 12 hours after the onset of headache, and 93% within the first 24 hours, but sensitivity falls off rapidly after the first 24 hours.

Patients at high risk for intracranial pathology, including HIV-positive individuals and cancer patients, should be imaged when presenting with new-onset headaches.

■ TREATMENT

HEADACHE DIARY

A headache diary can be a very useful tool in determining a headache trigger, be it environmental, food based, or even social. There are complex worksheets available that require the patient to keep very detailed records of each headache, but there is no evidence that this has any value greater than a simple headache log. Have the patient record very simply the date and time of the onset of headache, severity, any concurrent activity or food eaten if food is a suspected trigger, and treatment method, if used.

MEDICATION FOR ACUTE HEADACHES

NSAIDs: Benign exertional headaches are particularly responsive to indomethacin taken before the exertional activity or to other medications such as Rofecoxib and even aspirin. Caution should be used in the patient with gastrointestinal pathologies, in which case either switching to a cox-2 inhibitor such as Celebrex or adding a proton-pump inhibitor may be useful. Cox-2 inhibitors should not be used in patients with a cardiac history.

Acetaminophen: Acetaminophen is considered to be less effective than NSAID treatment, but it is well tolerated and can be useful as an adjunct therapy.

Triptans: These are considered first-line treatment of moderate to severe migraine pain. Their use is contraindicated in patients with coronary artery disease.

Ergots: These are less specific in their biochemical mode of action compared with triptans, and they have a resultant larger side-effect profile. Despite this, some patients find them to be more effective in acute migraine treatment than the triptans.

Barbiturates: Barbiturates should not form the mainstay of headache treatment, but can be very effective as an acute abortive medication when other treatments have failed.

Narcotics: The use of opioids in the treatment of headaches is one that has been widely discussed over the years. Current thinking holds that there is a limited place for the use of narcotic pain medication in the treatment of headache disorders, limiting its use to situations when all other abortive treatments have failed. They are appropriate only for short-term and intermittent use. Caution should be used when treating cluster headaches as narcotics may expedite transformation of episodic cluster headaches to chronic cluster headaches.

Perriactin (cyproheptadine): It is used in the treatment of migraine attacks and other similar headaches. It is not fully understood how it works in this condition. However, in addition to blocking the actions of histamine, cyproheptadine is also known to block the action of serotonin, which is known to be involved in migraine. Perriactin may be helpful for people whose headaches are not relieved by other migraine treatments.

Corticosteroids: These are extremely effective in terminating a cluster headache cycle and in preventing immediate headache recurrence. High-dose prednisone with an extended taper is prescribed. It is recommended that prophylactic headache treatment be started simultaneously. The mechanism of action in cluster headaches is still subject to speculation.

PROPHYLACTIC MEDICATIONS

Calcium channel blockers: These are effective prophylactic agents for both migraine and cluster headaches. They can be combined relatively easily with other prophylactic medications if required. Of the calcium channel blockers, verapamil is most frequently used.

Lithium: It is used in the treatment of cluster headaches, presumably due to their cyclical nature. Although responses vary, lithium has been shown to effectively prevent cluster headaches, particularly in its more chronic forms, and is considered a first-line treatment.

Anticonvulsants: There are data from a number of controlled studies that have found anticonvulsants to be effective in the prophylaxis of migraine and cluster headaches, though the mechanism of action remains unclear. Topiramate and divalproex are FDA approved for prophylaxis and with good clinical evidence to their efficacy. These drugs seem to be more effective with longer duration of treatment.

Tricyclic antidepressants: These are first-line therapy in the prophylaxis of migraines. There are a number of small studies that have demonstrated efficacy. The most common tricyclic antidepressant used is amitriptyline at low doses.

Beta-blockers: These are considered first-line therapy for migraines. Caution should be used when treating cluster headaches as they may worsen bradycardia occurring during the cluster attack.

Butterbur: It is a common plant that in clinical trials has been shown to be effective in the prevention of migraine headaches. It should be noted that the butterbur plant is hepatotoxic, carcinogenic, and teratogenic.

Magnesium: Magnesium deficiency is well documented in some people with migraine and cluster-type headaches. Magnesium is poorly absorbed and has a tendency to cause diarrhea; the slow release forms may be better tolerated and have greater bioavailability. Oral supplementation may be needed for more than 1 month before benefits are noticed.

LIFESTYLE MODIFICATION

Headache diet: Certain chemicals in foods can either act as a trigger for headaches or reduce the threshold for developing a headache (Table 21.4). These chemicals include tyramine, sulfites, monosodium glutamate (MSG), and aspartame. Reducing the amount consumed of these substances can significantly reduce the frequency of headaches and sometimes result in complete resolution.

Migraine headaches may respond to a low tyramine diet. Tyramine is not added to foods; it is produced in foods from the natural breakdown of the amino acid tyrosine. Tyramine levels increase in foods when they are aged, fermented, stored for long periods, or are not fresh.

Table 21.4 ■ **COMMON MIGRAINE TRIGGERS**

Specific food triggers	Aged cheese (and other foods, such as smoked fish, that are high in tyramine)
	Alcohol and red wine
	Artificial sweeteners
	Chocolate
	Citrus fruits
	Coffee, tea, and cola
	Monosodium glutamate (MSG)
	Nitrates in cured and processed meats (hot dogs and lunch meats)
	Nuts and peanut butter
	Salty foods
	Excess sugar
Environmental	Bright or glaring lights
	Flashing lights or screens
	Odors such as perfume
	Pollution and smog
	Barometric pressure changes
Physical factors	Dietary habits such as skipping meals and fasting
	Changes in sleep patterns including sleeping too little or too much
	Overexertion
	Becoming overly tired
	Dehydration
	Hormonal changes

Exercise: Regular exercise, such as walking three times a week, may reduce the frequency and intensity of certain headache syndromes. Excessive exercise, however, can be a trigger for headaches such as cluster headaches, in which case moderation is advised.

Yoga, tai chi, and other kinds of mindfulness-training exercise are now being recognized as having the additional value of reducing stress and increasing cognitive function—a symptom of many of the headache syndromes.

Smoking: Cigarette smoking can affect circulation, increasing the risk of headaches and other pain syndromes.

Nutrition: Healthy eating is especially important to ensure a balanced diet. Mindful eating includes avoidance of known triggering foods. In addition, as low blood sugar can act as a trigger for headaches, consistency is important.

Alcohol: Alcohol may worsen headaches and act as a trigger to many of the headache syndromes.

OTHER TREATMENT PROCEDURES

Botulinum toxin injections have been shown to be effective in the management of migraines. In other headache syndromes, the success rate is more limited. Greater occipital nerve block may be beneficial in aborting cluster headaches. Nerve blocks, ablative procedures, and brain stimulation are options for cases of refractory headache syndromes and have been used with varying success.

APPENDIX

USEFUL WEBSITES

Alzheimer's Association
www.alz.org

Alzheimer's Foundation of America
www.alzfdn.org

American Academy of Neurology
www.aan.com

American Diabetes Association
www.diabetes.org

International Headache Society
www.ihs-headache.org

International Parkinson and Movement Disorder Society
www.movementdisorders.org/MDS.htm

Muscular Dystrophy Organization
mda.org

National Multiple Sclerosis Foundation
www.nationalmssociety.org

National Parkinson Foundation
www.parkinson.org

BIBLIOGRAPHY

American Association of Neurological Surgeons. (2003). *Movement disorders: Patient education.* Retrieved from http://www.aans.org/Patient%20Information/Conditions%20and%20Treatments/Movement%20Disorders.aspx

Biller, J., Gruener, G., & Brazis, P. (2011). *DeMeyer's the neurologic examination: A programmed text* (6th ed.). New York, NY: The McGraw-Hill Companies.

Bisdorf, A., Von Brevern, M., Lempert, T., & Newman-Toker, D. E. (2009). Classification of vestibular symptoms: Towards and international classification of vestibular disorders [Electronic]. *Journal of Vestibular Research, 19*(1–2), 1–13.

Campbell, W. W. (2005). *DeJong's the neurologic examination* (6th ed.). Philadelphia, PA: Lippincott Williams & Wilkins.

Cooper, G. (2013). *Nonoperative treatment of osteoporotic compression fractures overview of osteoporotic compression fractures.* Retrieved from http://emedicine.medscape.com/article/325872-overview

Corey-Bloom, J., & David, R. B. (2009). *Clinical adult neurology* (3rd ed.). New York, NY: Demos Medical Publishing.

Cramer, G. D., & Darby, S. A. (2005). *Basic and clinical anatomy of the spine, spinal cord, and ANS* (2nd ed.). St Louis, MO: Elsevier Mosby.

Dogu, O., Sevim, S., Camdeviren, H., Sasmaz, T., Bugdayci, R., Aral, M., … Louis, E. D. (2003). Prevalence of essential tremor: Door-to-door neurologic exams in Mersin Province, Turkey [Electronic]. *Neurology, 61*(12), 1804–1806.

Doty, R. L. (2009). The olfactory system and its disorders [Electronic]. *Seminars in Neurology, 29*(1), 74–81.

Duby, J. J., Campbell, R. K., Setter, S. M., White, J. R., & Rasmussen, K. A. (2004). Diabetic neuropathy: An intensive review [Electronic]. *American Journal of Health-System Pharmacy, 61*(2), 160–173.

Edwards, M., & Deuschl, G. (2013). Tremor syndromes. *Continuum: Lifelong Learning in Neurology, 19*(5), 1213–1224.

Ehrenhaus, M. P. (2014). *Abducens nerve palsy*. Retrieved from http://emedicine.medscape.com/article/1198383-overview

Fasano, A., & Bloem, B. (2013). Movement disorders. *Continuum: Lifelong Learning in Neurology, 19*(5), 1344–1382.

Galluzzi, K. E. (2007). Managing neuropathic pain. *Journal of the American Osteopathic Association, 107*(Suppl. 6), ES39–ES48.

Gilron, I., Peter, C., Watson, N., Cahill, C. M., & Moulin, D. E. (2006). Neuropathic pain: A practical guide for the clinician [Electronic]. *Canadian Medical Association Journal, 175*(3), 265–275.

Goldberg, S. (2004). *The four-minute neurologic exam*. Miami, FL: Medmaster.

Green, P., Rohling, M. L., Iverson, G. L., & Gervais, R. O. (2003). Relationships between olfactory discrimination and head injury severity. *Brain Injury, 17*(6), 479–496. doi:10.1080/0269905031000070242

Guarantors of Brain. (2000). *Aids to the examination of the peripheral nervous system* (4th ed.). Philadelphia, PA: Elsevier Saunders.

Hoppenfeld, S. (1976). *Physical examination of the spine and extremities*. Upper Saddle River, NJ: Prentice Hall.

Mazzoni, P., & Rowland, L. P. (2001). *Merritt's neurology handbook*. Philadelphia, PA: Lippincott Williams & Wilkins.

Miller, A. E. (Editor-in-Chief). (2012a). Dementia. *Continuum: Lifelong Learning in Neurology, 19*(2), 372–424.

Miller, A. E. (Editor-in-Chief). (2012b). Headache. *Continuum: Lifelong Learning in Neurology, 18*(4), 753–835.

Miller, A. E. (Editor-in-Chief). (2012c). Neuro-otology. *Continuum: Lifelong Learning in Neurology, 18*(5), 1041–1101.

Miller, A. E. (Editor-in-Chief). (2012d). Peripheral neuropathy. *Continuum: Lifelong Learning in Neurology, 18*(1), 60–160.

Mori, M., Kuwabara, S., Fukutake, T., Yuki, N., & Hattori, T. (2001). Clinical features and prognosis of Miller Fisher syndrome [Electronic]. *Neurology, 56*(8), 1104–1106.

Rajput, A., Robinson, C. A., & Rajput, A. H. (2004). Essential tremor course and disability: A clinicopathologic study of 20 cases. *Neurology, 62*(6), 932–936

Reeves, A. G., & Swenson, R. S. (2008). Disorders of the nervous system [Electronic]. Retrieved from http://www.dartmouth.edu/~dons/index.html

Rohkamm, R. (2004). *Color atlas of neurology*. New York, NY: Thieme.

Ropper, A. H., & Samuels, M. A. (2009). *Adams and Victor's principles of neurology* (9th ed.). New York, NY: The McGraw-Hill Companies.

Rowen, A. J., & Tolunsky, E. (2003). *Primer of EEG*. Philadelphia, PA: Butterworth Heinemann.

Saper, J. R., Silberstein, S., Gordon, C. D., Hamel, R. L., & Swidan, S. (1999). *Handbook of headache management: A practical guide to diagnosis and treatment of head, neck and facial pain* (2nd ed.). Baltimore, MD: Lippincott Williams & Wilkins.

Sheik, Z. A., & Hutcheson, K. A. (2014). *Trochlear nerve palsy*. Retrieved from http://emedicine.medscape.com/article/1200187-overview

Silberstein, S. D., Lipton, R. B., & Goadsby, P. J. (2002) *Headache in clinical practice* (2nd ed.). London, UK: Martin Dunitz.

Smorto, M. P., & Basmajian, J. V. (1980). *Neuromotor examination of the limbs: A photographic atlas*. Baltimore, MD: Williams and Wilkins.

Task Force for the Diagnosis and Management of Syncope of the European Society of Cardiology (ESC). (2009). Guidelines for the diagnosis and management of syncope (version 2009) [Electronic]. *European Heart Journal, 30*(21), 2631–2671.

Thompson, T. L., & Amedee, R. (2009). Vertigo: A review of common peripheral and central vestibular disorders. *The Ochsner Journal, 9*(1), 20–26.

Tripathi, M., & Vibha, D. (2009). Reversible dementias. *Indian Journal of Psychiatry, 51*(1), S53–S55.

Wherrett, J. R. (2008). The role of the neurologic examination in the diagnosis and categorization of dementia. *Geriatrics and Aging, 11*(4), 203–208.

Wilson-Pauwells, L., Akesson, E. J., Steweart, P. A., & Spacey, S. D. (2002). *Cranial nerves in health and disease* (2nd ed.). Hamilton, ON: B.C. Decker.

Index

abducens nerve (CN VI), 30, 209
abstract reasoning, assessment
    of, 19
accessory nerve (CN XI), 48–49
acetaminophen, for acute
    headaches, 234
Achilles reflex, 85
acquired peripheral neuropathies,
    172–173
acute headaches, medication for,
    234–235
acute traumatic compression
    fractures, 159–161
adiadochokinesia, 108
afferent pupillary defect, 23
agnosia, 20
alcohol, tobacco and illicit drug
    use, in history taking, 9
alcoholic dementia, 205
alcoholic neuropathy, 176–177
Alzheimer's disease, 199–202, 206,
    219–220
amitriptyline
    for headaches, 235
    for peripheral neuropathy, 180
ampyra (dalfampridine), for gait
    disturbance, 220
anal wink reflex, 90
anarthria. *See* dysarthria
anesthetic skin, 72
ankle-foot orthosis (AFO), 221

antalgic gait, 96–97
anticholinergic medications, for
    vertigo, 138
anticonvulsants, for
    headaches, 235
antiseizure medications,
    for peripheral
    polyneuropathy, 179
aphasia. *See* dysphasia
aphonia. *See* dysphonia
apraxia, 20
arm swing, 93
associated symptoms, in history
    taking, 7–8
ataxia, 100, 217
    cerebellar, 100, 102
    like findings, etiologies of, 110
    sensory, 102
ataxic tremor. *See* intention tremor
axonal degeneration, 172

balance, 94–95
barbiturates, for acute
    headaches, 234
Bell's palsy, 41, 42
benign paroxysmal positional
    vertigo (BPPV), 127–129
benzodiazepines, for vertigo, 138
beta-blockers, for headaches, 235
bicep muscle, 56, 57
biceps reflex, 82

binocular diplopia, 208, 210–213
botulinum toxin injections, for
    migraines, 237
brachioradialis reflex, 84
bursitis, 153–154
burst fractures, 161–162
butterbur, for headaches, 235

cadence, 92
calcium channel blockers, for
    headaches, 235
caloric stimulation test, 45–46
canalith repositioning
    procedures, 135
capsaicin, for peripheral
    polyneuropathy, 179
carbamazepine (Tegretol), 179
cataracts, 26–27, 208, 213
cauda equine syndrome
    bladder dysfunction in, 166
    spinal cord compression and,
        164–167
center of gravity, 92
central nervous system lesions,
    212–213
cerebellar ataxia, 100, 102
cerebellar tremor. *See* intention
    tremor
cervical spondolytic myelopathy,
    65–66
chelated gadolinium, 118
chief complaint, 4–5
cholinesterase inhibitors, for
    Alzheimer disease, 206
chronic dementias, 198–199
chronic inflammatory
    demyelinating
    polyneuropathy
    (CIDP), 192
circumduction. *See* Trendelenburg
    gait
clasp-knife phenomenon, 53
classic essential tremor, 146
clonus, 85–88

cluster headache, 229–230
cogwheeling, 53
color desaturation testing, 27
complete metabolic panel
    (CMP), 178
compression fractures, 158–162
computed tomography scans,
    115–117
congenital myopathy, 185–187
conus medullaris, 164
coordination testing, 105–111
    interpretation of, 110–111
    testing patient, 108–109
    tests used, 105–108
corneal reflex, 39, 88–90
cortical sensation, 76–77
    extinction, 77
    graphesthesia, 76–77
    stereognosia, 76
corticosteroids, 191
    for acute headaches, 234–235
    for metabolic myopathies, 187
    for neuromuscular disease,
        194–195
    for vertigo, 138
cranial nerves
    VIII. *See* vestibulocochlear nerve
    XI. *See* accessory nerve
    extraocular eye movement, 34
    V. *See* trigeminal nerve
    IV. *See* trochlear nerve
    fourth nerve palsy, 34–35, 209
    IX. *See* glossopharyngeal nerve
    I. *See* olfactory nerve
    palsies, 30–35, 208–210
    VII. *See* facial nerve
    VI. *See* abducens nerve
    sixth nerve palsy, 35, 209–210
    X. *See* vagus nerve
    third nerve palsy, 32, 33, 209
    III. *See* oculomotor nerve
    XII. *See* hypoglossal nerve
    II. *See* optic nerve
    visual fields testing, 34

cross-checking symptomology, 7
CT angiography, 117
CT myelogram, 117
cyclosporine (Neoral,
        Sandimmune), 195
Cymbalta, 180

decreased sensation, 72
deep tendon reflexes, 80–88
degenerative osteoarthritis. *See*
        cervical spondolytic
        myelopathy
deltoid muscle, 56
dementia, 197–206
    additional testing, 204
    characteristics of, 197
    clinical approach, 197–199
    criterion-based diagnosis,
        199–203
        Alzheimer's disease,
        199–202
        vascular dementia, 202
    diagnosis of, 197, 203
    etiologies of reversible, 198
    imaging studies, 204
    important labs, 204
    medication for, 206
    mixed, 202
    questions to ask patient, 203
    risk, prevention and treatment,
        204–206
        exercise, 205
        nutrition, 205
        sleep, 205–206
dermatomal sensory patterns,
        69–72
diabetes mellitus
    diplopia and, 212
    gait disturbance and, 220–221
    peripheral neuropathy and, 54,
        69, 171–172, 173
diabetic foot drop, 221
diabetic peripheral neuropathy,
        173, 180, 212, 220

*Diagnostic and Statistical Manual
        of Mental Disorders*
        (DSM), 199
    for Alzheimer disease,
        199–202
    for vascular dementia, 202
diplopia, 31, 207–215
    binocular, 208
        testing for, 210–213
    cannot-miss causes of, 213
    imaging techniques, 214
    important labs, 214
    monocular, 207–208
        testing for, 213
    nerve palsies, 208–210
        fourth nerve palsy, 209
        sixth nerve palsy, 209–210
        third nerve palsy, 209
    questions to ask patients, 214
    testing for, 210–213
    treatment, 215
direct questions, in history taking, 6
diuretics, for vertigo, 138
divalproex, for headaches, 235
Dix–Hallpike maneuver,
        128–129, 134
dizziness, 126, 127–128
dorsiflexor strength, 62
double vision. *See* diplopia
drug-induced tremors, 146–147
Duchenne muscular dystrophy, 188
dying-back phenomenon. *See*
        axonal degeneration
dysarthria, 16
dysphasia, 16
dysphonia, 14–16

edrophonium (Tensilon) testing, 190
Effexor, 180
electromyogram, 179, 193–194
electromyography, nerve
        conduction velocity studies
        and, 118–121, 191
enhanced physiologic tremor, 142

epidural spinal cord
compression, 165
Epley maneuver, 128, 135,
136–137
ergots, for acute headaches, 234
erythrocyte sedimentation rate
(ESR), 178
essential tremor, 146
exertional headaches, 230
extensor hallucis longus (EHL)
muscle, 62, 63
extinction, 77
extraocular eye movement, 34

FABERE test, 155
facial nerve, 40–42
acoustic reflex, 41
Bell's palsy, 41, 42
facial expressions, muscles
of, 41
familial essential tremor, 146
family history, 9
fatigue, 184
festination gait, 98–99
fifth cervical nerve (C5), 56
finger flexor reflex. See Hoffman's
reflex
finger-to-nose testing, 105, 106,
108, 109
finger-to-nose-to-finger, 105–106
fingers
adduction, 60
flexion, 59
fluoroscopy, 115
foot dorsiflexion, 221
foot drop, 217
foot tapping, 108
fourth nerve palsy, 34–35, 209
freezing of gait (FOG), 99–100
frontal gait disorder, 219
fund of knowledge, assessment of
general, 19–20
fundoscopic exam, 25–27

gabapentin (Neurontin), 179
Gaenslen sign, 156
gag reflex, 90
gag response, 47–48
gait
antalgic, 96–97
ataxia, 100
examination of, 92–93
arm swing, 93
balance, 94–95
cadence, 92
center of gravity, 92
length of a step, 92
turning problems, 93
width of gait, 92
festination, 98–99
freezing of, 99–100
hemiplegic, 97, 99
hypokinetic, 98, 101
as measure of functional capacity, 95–96
motor component of, 91–92
myopathic, 97
naming neurologic, 96–103
phases of, 92
provocative testing of, 94
scissors, 102–103
sensory component of, 91
spastic, 97, 100
steppage, 97–98, 101
Trendelenburg, 97, 98
gait disturbance, 217–222
Alzheimer disease, 219–220
causes of, 217
clinical approach, 217–221
diabetes, 220–221
etiologies of, 218
imaging techniques, 222
important labs, 221
multiple sclerosis, 220
Parkinson's disease, 219
questions to ask patient, 221
treatment, 222

assistive devices and orthod-
    ics, 222
physical therapy, 222
spasticity, 222
gastroc strength, 94
gastrocnemius muscle, 64, 94
glomerular filtration rate
    (GFR), 118
glossopharyngeal nerve (CN IX),
    47–48
graphesthesia, 76–77
Graves's disease, 211–212
Guillain-Barré syndrome (GBS),
    191–192, 212

H1-receptor antagonists, for
    vertigo, 138
hand-slap test, 106–107, 108–109
head pain, clinical approaches to,
    223–231
head thrust test. *See* unilateral
    head impulse test
headache diary, 233
headache diet, 236
headaches, 223–238
    cannot-miss causes of, 225–228
    clinical approaches to, 223–231
    cluster, 229–230
    exertional, 230
    imaging, 232–233
    laboratory tests for, 232
    medication overuse, 231
    migraines, 223, 229
    primary causes of, 224
    questions to ask patient,
        231–232
    rebound, 231
    tension, 230
    thunderclap, 231
    treatment, 233–237
        botulinum toxin injections
            for, 237
        headache diary, 233

lifestyle modification,
    236–237
medication for acute
    headaches, 234–235
prophylactic medications, 235
heel-to-shin testing, 107, 109
heel walking, 61–62, 64
hemiplegic gait, 97, 99
herpes, 39
higher order sensory testing.
    See cortical sensation
hippus, 22
history taking, essential elements
    of, 3–4
    cross-checking symptomology, 7
    formatting history of present
        illness, 4–9
        aggravating/relieving
            factors, 7–8
        associated symptoms, 7–8
        chief complaint, 4–5
        determining onset, 7
        occupational, psychosocial
            and family history, 8–9
        past medical history, 8
    listen, 3–4
    value of thorough patient his-
        tory, 9–10
HIV, 177–178
Hoffman's reflex, 85
Holme's tremor. *See* rubral tremor
horizontal double vision, 210
hyperreflexia, 81
hypertonia, 53
hypertrophy, 51–52
hypoglossal nerve (CN XII), 49–50
hypokinetic gait, 98, 101
hyporeflexia, 82
hypothyroidism, 173
hypotonia, 53

iliopsoas muscle, 60
immediate memory, 18

immunosuppressants, for
    weakness, 195
inclusion-body myositis, 187
induced weakness, 183
inflammatory myopathies, 187
injections
    botulinum toxin, 237
    for low back pain, 169
intention tremor, 146
International Headache Society, 223
internuclear ophthalmoplegia
    (INO), 211
intervertebral disk protrusions, 164
iodinated contrast dye, 115
IVIg, 195

kyphosis, 159, 161

labyrinthitis, 133–134
Lambert–Eaton myasthenic
    syndrome (LEMS), 191
lead-pipe resistance, 53
length of a step, 92
level of consciousness, assessment
    of, 14
Lhermitte's sign, 90
lidocaine patch, for peripheral
    polyneuropathy, 179
lifestyle modifications
    for headache, 236
    for peripheral neuropathy,
        180–181
light touch, testing, 72–73
lithium, for cluster headaches, 235
long-term memory, assessment
    of, 19
low back pain, 151–169
    cauda equina syndrome, 164–167
    clinical approach to, 151–152
    compression fractures, 158–162
        acute traumatic, 159–161
        burst, 161–162
        osteoporotic, 159
    imaging studies, 167–168
    laboratory tests, 167

muscle strain and sprain, 152
    nerve root compression, 163–164
    pars defect, 162–163
    piriformis syndrome, 157
    questions to ask patient, 167
    sacroiliac joints, 154–156
        Gaenslen sign, 156
        Patrick test, 155
    spinal cord compression,
        164–167
    straight leg raise test, 164
    treatment, 168–169
        patient-controlled modalities,
            168
        provider-prescribed modali-
            ties, 168–169
    trochanteric bursitis, 153–154
    worrisome symptoms, evaluat-
        ing, 166
lower extremity coordination
    testing, 107
lower motor neuron system, 66–67
lumbar strains, 152

magnesium, for headaches, 235
magnetic resonance angiogram
    (MRA), 135
magnetic resonance imaging,
    117–118
managing sensitive aspects of
    symptoms, 6
memantine (Namenda), for
    Alzheimer's disease, 206
memory
    assessment of, 17–19
        ability to recount recent
            events, 18–19
        immediate recall, 18
        long-term memory, 19
    definition, 17
    remote, 17
Ménière's disease, 130, 133
mental status testing, 11–20
    abstract reasoning, assessment
        of, 19

calculation, assessment of, 20
formal tests for, 11–14
fund of knowledge, assessment of general, 19–20
level of consciousness, assessment of, 14, 15
memory, assessment of, 17–19
object recognition, assessment of, 20
orientation, assessment of, 16–17
speech, assessment of, 14–16
voluntary movement, assessment of, 20
metabolic myopathies, 187
metformin, 118
migraines, 223, 229
aura, 229
characteristics of, 229
triggering factors of, 229, 236
Miller Fisher syndrome (MFS), 212
Mini-Mental State Examination (MMSE), 11–12
mixed dementia, 202
modified Glasgow Coma Scale (GCS), 14, 15
monocular diplopia, 207–208
causes of, 213
testing for, 213
mononeuropathy, 53
monosynaptic reflexes, 80
Montreal Cognitive Assessment Test (MoCA), 11–12, 14
motor neurons, 51
motor neuropathy, 221
motor strength, testing, 51–67
motor system dysfunction, 66–67
muscle function, 51–52
myelopathy, 65–66
nerve root evaluation, 54–64
peripheral motor strength, 53–54
motor system dysfunction, 66–67
multiple sclerosis (MS), 220
diplopia in, 210–211

muscle function, 51–52
strength, 53, 54
tone, 53
trophic state, 51–52
muscle strain, 152
muscle tightness. *See* spasticity
muscle tone, 53
muscle weakness, 188, 190, 191, 217, 220
muscles' trophic state, 51–52
muscular dystrophies, 188
myasthenia gravis (MG), 188–191, 211
symptoms, 188, 190
testing for, 190
treatment for, 191
mycophenolate mofetil (Cellcept), 195
myelopathy, 65–66
myopathic gait, 97, 98, 217
myotatic reflex. *See* deep tendon reflexes
myotomes
cervical nerve roots and, 55
lumbar nerve roots and, 55

narcotics, for acute headaches, 234
nerve conduction velocity (NCV) studies, 118–121
nerve root compression, 163–164
nerve root evaluation, 54–64
C5, 56
C6, 57
C7, 58–59
C8, 59
cervical nerve roots and myotomes, 55
L1, 2, and 3, 60
L2, 3, and 4, 60–61, 62
L4, 61–62, 63
L5, 62, 63
lumbar nerve roots and myotomes, 55
S1 and S2, 64
T1, 60

neuromuscular junction diseases, 188–192
  chronic inflammatory demyelin-ating polyneuropathy, 192
  Guillain-Barré syndrome, 191–192
  Lambert–Eaton myasthenic syndrome, 191
  myasthenia gravis, 188–191
neuropathic gait. *See* steppage gait
neuropathies
  basic characteristics of, 174–175
  of poor nutrition, 176–177
nonsteroidal anti-inflammatory drugs (NSAIDs), 154
  for acute headaches, 234
  for low back pain, 168
nystagmus, 34, 46, 129–130, 137, 210

object recognition, assessment of, 20
occupational history, 8–9
oculomotor nerve (CN III), 30
  eye movement and, 209
olfactory nerve (CN I), 21–22
open-ended questions, in history taking, 5
opioids, for peripheral polyneuropathy, 179
optic nerve (CN II), 22–27
  afferent pupillary defect, 23
  color desaturation, 27
  fundoscopic exam, 25–27
  pupillary light reflex, 22
  visual acuity, 25
  visual fields, 23–25
oral steroids, for low back pain, 168
orientation, assessment of, 16–17
  to persons, 16–17
  to place, 17
  to time/date/season, 17
orthostatic tremor, 147

osteoporotic compression fractures, 159
over-the-counter analgesics, for peripheral polyneuropathy, 179
oxycodone (Roxicodone), 179

pain
  low back. *See* low back pain
  sensation, 73
  and temperature sensation, 73
palsy, 30–35
paratonia (gegenhalten), 53
Parkinson's disease (PD), 98, 219
Parkinsonian tremor, 146
pars defect, 162–163
patellar reflex, 85
pathologies, imaging techniques for common, 113
Patrick test. *See* FABERE test
perceived weakness
  definition, 183
  true weakness versus, 184
Percocet, 179
peripheral motor neuropathy, 53–54
peripheral neuropathy, 171–181
  alcoholic neuropathy, 176–177
  clinical approach, 172–177
  diabetes, 173
  electromyogram testing, 179
  HIV and venereal diseases, 177, 178
  hypothyroidism, 173
  imaging, 179
  important labs, 178
  neuropathy of poor nutrition, 176–177
  questions to ask patient, 178
  toxins, 177
  treatment, 179–181
    lifestyle modifications, 180–181
    medications, 179–180
    therapies, 180

peripheral polyneuropathy, 178
peripheral sensory changes, 70
perriactin (cyproheptadine), for
    acute headaches, 234
phenytoin (Dilantin), 179
phonation, 47
physical therapy (PT)
    for gait disturbance, 222
    for low back pain, 168–169
    for neuromuscular disease, 194
    for vertigo, 138–139
physiologic tremor, 142
pill-rolling-type tremor, 146
pinprick testing, 73
pins-and-needles numbness, 72
piriformis syndrome, 157
plain x-ray films, 114
plantar reflex, 88
polyneuropathy, 53
polysynaptic reflexes, 80
pregabalin (Lyrica), 179
present illness, history of, 4–9
presyncope, 126
primary headaches, 223
primary myopathies, 185–188
    congenital myopathy, 185–187
    inflammatory myopathies, 187
    metabolic myopathies, 187
    muscular dystrophies, 188
prophylactic medications, for
        acute headaches, 235
proprioception, 69
    definition, 74
    loss of, 74–75
    tests for, 75
psychogenic tremor, 147
pupillary light reflex, 22
pupillary reflex, 32

quadriceps muscles, 60–61, 62

radiation exposure, 115–116
rapid alternating hand movement
    test. See hand-slap test

rapid foot tapping. See heel to-shin
        testing
rapid toe-tapping, 109
rebound headaches, 231
reflexes, 79–90
    Achilles reflex, 85
    anal wink reflex, 90
    biceps, 82, 83
    brachioradialis, 84
    clonus, 85–88
    corneal, 88–90
    deep tendon, 80–88
    gag reflex, 90
    grading table, 82
    Lhermitte's sign, 90
    monosynaptic, 80
    in neurologic examination, 79
    patellar, 85
    plantar, 88
    polysynaptic, 80
    superficial, 88–90
    triceps, 82–83
remote memory, 17
reversible dementia, 198, 205
Rinne test, 43–44
rituximab (Rituxan), 195
Romberg test, 94, 134
rubral tremor, 146

sacroiliac joints (SI joints), 154–155
sacroiliitis, 154–155
Savella, 180
scissors gait, 102–103
segmental demyelination, 172
sensation, testing, 69–77
    cortical sensation, 76–77
    dermatomal sensory patterns,
        69–72
    light touch, testing, 72–73
    pinprick testing, 73
    proprioception, 69, 74–75
    skin sensations, 69
    temperature, 73
    vibration, 74

sensory ataxia, 102
6-Item Cognitive Impairment Test
    (6CIT), 11–13, 14
sixth nerve palsy, 35, 209–210
skew deviation, 212–213
skin sensations, 69
Snellen chart, 25, 26
SNRIs, for peripheral
    polyneuropathy, 180
spastic gait, 97, 100
spasticity, 217, 220, 222
speech, assessment of, 14–16
    dysarthria, 16
    dysphasia, 16
    dysphonia, 14–16
spinal cord compression, 164–167
sprain, 152
steppage gait, 97–98, 101
stereognosia, 76
sternocleidomastoid muscles,
    testing, 48–49
steroid myositis, 195
straight leg raise test, 164
stretch reflex. *See* deep tendon
    reflexes
suicide headaches. *See* cluster
    headaches
superficial reflexes, 88
    anal wink reflex, 90
    corneal reflex, 88–90
    gag reflex, 90
    Lhermitte's sign, 90
    plantar reflex, 88
swallow, 47
syncope, 126
systemic-illness tremor, 146–147

tacrolimus (Prograf), 195
tension headaches, 230
third nerve palsy, 32, 33, 209
thunderclap headache, 231
topiramate (Topamax), 179, 235
touch sensation, 72–73
toxins, 177
tramadol (Ultram ER), 179

transcutaneous electrical nerve
    stimulation (TENS), 180
trapezius, testing, 48–49
traumatic brain injury (TBI), 21–22
tremor, 141–150
    basic characteristics of,
        143–145
    clinical approach to, 142–148
    definition, 141
    drug-induced, 146–147
    enhanced physiologic, 142
    essential, 146
    imaging studies, 148
    intention, 146
    laboratory tests, 148
    orthostatic, 147
    Parkinsonian tremor, 146
    pathophysiology of, 141
    physiologic, 142
    psychogenic, 147
    questions to ask patient,
        147–148
    size of, 141–142
    speed of, 141
    systemic illness, 146–147
    treatment, 149
Trendelenburg gait. *See* myopathic
    gait
triceps muscle, 58–59
triceps reflex, 82–83
tricyclic antidepressants
    for headaches, 235
    for peripheral
        polyneuropathy, 180
trigeminal nerve (CN V), 37–39
    corneal reflex, 39
    herpes, 39
    motor, 38
    testing sensory component
        of, 38
    trigeminal neuralgia, 39
trigeminal neuralgia, 39
trigger points, 169
triptans, for acute headaches, 234
trochanteric bursitis, 153–154

trochlear nerve (CN IV), 30, 209
true weakness, 183
   definition, 183
   fatigue versus, 184
   perceived weakness versus, 184
turning problems, 93
20/15 vision, 25
20/20 vision, 25
20/40 vision, 25
20/200 vision, 25
tyramine, migraine headaches
   and, 236

unilateral head impulse test,
   45, 46
unsteadiness, 126
upper motor neuron system,
   66–67

vagus nerve (CN X), 47–48
vascular dementia, 202
venereal disease, 178
vertical double vision, 210
vertigo, 125–139
   benign paroxysmal positional
      vertigo, 128
   causes of, 125
   clinical approaches to, 126–134
   definitions of, 125, 126
   Dix–Hallpike maneuver,
      128–129, 134
   home remedies, 139
   imaging studies, 135
   laboratory tests, 134
   labyrinthitis, 133–134
   medications, 138
   Ménière's disease, 130, 133
   physical therapy, 138–139
   questions to ask patient, 134
   special testing, 134–135

treatment
   Epley maneuver, 136–137
   repositioning procedures, 135
   vestibular neuronitis, 133–134
vestibular neuronitis, 133–134
vestibulocochlear nerve (CN VIII),
   42–46
   auditory system, 43
   caloric stimulation test, 45–46
   unilateral head impulse test,
      45, 46
   vestibular system, 45
   Weber and Rinne tests, 43–44
vibration sensation, 74
Vicodin, 179
visual acuity, 25
visual fields, 22, 23–25, 34
voluntary movement, assessment
   of, 20

Wallerian degeneration, 172
weakness, 183–195
   arising from central nervous
      system, 184, 185
   biopsies, 194
   clinical approach, 183–192
   important labs, 193
   induced, 183
   neuromuscular junction
      diseases, 188–192
   perceived, 183
   primary myopathies, 185–188
   questions to ask patient, 192–193
   treatment
      dietary changes, 194
      exercise, 194
      medications, 194–195
   true, 183
Weber test, 43–44
width of gait, 92

Printed in the United States
By Bookmasters